Phototherapy in the Newborn: *An Overview*

COMMITTEE ON PHOTOTHERAPY IN THE NEWBORN
Division of Medical Sciences
Assembly of Life Sciences
National Research Council

Edited by
GERARD B. ODELL, M.D.
ROBERT SCHAFFER, PH.D.
ARTEMIS P. SIMOPOULOS, M.D.

NATIONAL ACADEMY OF SCIENCES
WASHINGTON, D.C. 1974

NOTICE The project that is the subject of this report was approved by the Governing Board of the National Research Council, acting in behalf of the National Academy of Sciences. Such approval reflects the Board's judgment that the project is of national importance and appropriate with respect to both the purposes and resources of the National Research Council.

The members of the committee selected to undertake this project and prepare this report were chosen for recognized scholarly competence and with due consideration for the balance of disciplines appropriate to the project. Responsibility for the detailed aspects of this report rests with that committee.

Each report issuing from a study committee of the National Research Council is reviewed by an independent group of qualified individuals according to procedures established and monitored by the Report Review Committee of the National Academy of Sciences. Distribution of the report is approved, by the President of the Academy, upon satisfactory completion of the review process.

This study was supported by the Maternal and Child Health Service, Health Services and Mental Health Administration, Department of Health, Education, and Welfare (Grant MC–R–110181–01–0).

Library of Congress Cataloging in Publication Data
Main entry under title:

Phototherapy in the newborn.

Contains selected papers from a symposium held Feb. 12–13, 1973, in Washington under the sponsorship of the Committee on Phototherapy in the Newborn, Assembly of Life Sciences and additional papers prepared by members of the committee.

Includes bibliographies.

1. Hyperbilirubinemia—Congresses. 2. Infants (Newborn)—Diseases—Congresses. 3. Phototherapy—Congresses. I. Odell, Gerard B., ed. II. Schaffer, Robert, 1920– ed. III. Simopoulos, Artemis P., ed. IV. Assembly of Life Sciences. Committee on Phototherapy in the Newborn. [DNLM: 1. Hyperbilirubinemia—In infancy and childhood. 2. Hyperbilirubinemia—Therapy. 3. Light—Therapeutic use. WB480 P575]

RJ276.P47 618.9'21'5 74–31207

ISBN 0–309–02313–0

Available from
Printing and Publishing Office, National Academy of Sciences
2101 Constitution Avenue, N.W., Washington, D.C. 20418

Printed in the United States of America

Preface

Instead of evolving smoothly in a progression of logical steps, medical advances often develop haltingly by a combination of empiricism, serendipity, and investigation. Studies of light as a therapeutic modality have followed this latter pattern over the past two decades. Only recently has there been systematic scientific investigation of some of the biological effects of light that may be relevant to health. The fact that a significant segment of our newborn population is receiving phototherapy each year for hyperbilirubinemia has given renewed emphasis to these studies.

A symposium on phototherapy was held in Washington, D.C., February 12 and 13, 1973, under the sponsorship of the Committee on Phototherapy in the Newborn. This volume includes selected papers presented at the symposium and additional papers prepared by various members of the Committee. It is intended to be of interest to photobiologists, photochemists, bioengineers, physicists, medical researchers, and clinicians.

The Committee hopes that this effort will provide additional perspective concerning this field and stimulate further investigation.

RICHARD E. BEHRMAN, M.D., *Chairman*
Committee on Phototherapy in the Newborn

Committee on Phototherapy in the Newborn

Richard E. Behrman, *Chairman*

Audrey K. Brown

Malcolm R. Currie

Leonard C. Harber

J. W. Hastings

Gerard B. Odell

Robert Schaffer

Richard B. Setlow

Thomas P. Vogl

Richard J. Wurtman

Contents

ROBERT J. ANDERSON, THOMAS P. VOGL, *and* JOHANNA S. SCHRUBEN

The Radiometry of Phototherapy

Introduction

The widespread use and apparent clinical acceptance of the technique of phototherapy for the treatment of neonatal hyperbilirubinemia have increased the necessity for accurately measuring the dosage of light administered. Although measurement of dosage is fundamental to both safety and efficacy of phototherapy, monitoring instruments appropriate for clinical use are not available. To further compound the problem, there is ambiguity and confusion in regard to the quantities that should be measured; the units and dimensions cited in the literature are generally either inconsistent or inaccurate, or both; and the instrumentation that is being used for radiometric measurements of phototherapy consists of a variety of instruments performing unrelated measurements, in part because the measurement procedures are not standardized.

This paper attempts to clarify the problem by reviewing the theory of radiometric and photometric measurements and units, defining what measurements need to be made, and specifying the characteristics to be sought in clinical radiometric instruments used for phototherapy.

Radiometry, Photometry, and Units

Strictly defined, light is radiation that is capable of producing visual response in human observers, but for many purposes it may be defined as

TABLE 1 Quantities in Radiometry and Photometry

	Radiometric			Photometric		
Dimension [a]	Quantity	Symbol	SI Units	Quantity	Symbol	SI Units
Q	Quantity of radiation	Q_e	Joule (J)	Quantity of light	Q	Lumen-second (lm·s)
W	Radiant flux	Φ_e	Watt (W)	Luminous flux	Φ	Lumen (lm)
W/A	Radiant emittance	M_e	Watts per square meter (W/m²)	Luminous emittance	M	Lumen per square meter (lm/m²)
W/A	Irradiation (irradiance)	E_e	Watts per square meter (W/m²)	Illumination (illuminance)	E	Lux (lx) [b]
W/Ω	Radiant intensity	I_e	Watts per steradian (W/sr)	Luminous intensity	I	Candela (cd)
$W/\Omega A$	Radiance	L_e	Watts per steradian per square meter ($W \cdot m^2 s^{-1}$)	Luminance	L	Candela per square meter (cd/m²)

[a] Q = energy, W = power, A = area, Ω = solid angle.
[b] Foot-candles in the English system of units (1 lx = 0.0929 ft-c).

electromagnetic radiation within a certain band of frequencies. Radiation in the regions immediately below or above the range of frequencies that can produce a visual response in human observers is called ultraviolet or infrared, respectively, and is frequently included in the term *light* in its broader sense.

Precise measurement is a fundamental principle of science, and the concepts upon which measurements are based are an important part of science. Unfortunately, in the measurement of light, the concepts have led to a vocabulary that is both ambiguous and confusing. We shall therefore review this vocabulary in terms of the standard accepted notation.

When the total power of the radiation is the quantity to be measured, the process of measurement is termed radiometry and the adjective *radiant* is used. If the measurement of power that is effective in producing a visual response in a human observer is of interest, the process is called photometry and the adjective *luminous* is used to describe the quantity measured. Hence, measurements in the visible region of the spectrum may be accomplished either by radiometry or photometry, with analogous quantities being denoted by the same symbol. However, the subscript "e" is used to identify the radiant quantity whenever there is danger of ambiguity. Although both radiometry and photometry measure quantities related to the power contained within a beam of light, photometry is related solely to the ability of that power to produce a visual response in the human eye. (Photometric measurements have no meaning in either the ultraviolet or infrared region of the spectrum.) Moreover, measurements in photometry are not absolute in the same sense as are those of radiometry, since there are individual variations in the ability of human observers to respond to visual stimuli, and it has therefore been necessary to arbitrarily define a "standard observer" for purposes of photometric measurements.

Table 1 summarizes the quantities used in radiometry and photometry. The symbols and units given are those of the International System of Units.[1–3, 8, 9, 13, 14]

RADIOMETRY

The basic quantity in radiometry is the radiant power traversing a surface defined arbitrarily in space. This power flow is called the radiant flux (ϕ_e). The unit of measurement of radiant flux is the watt. The total quantity of radiation that is passed through the surface is the time integral of the radiant flux and is measured in units of watt-seconds (joules).

The radiant flux impinging on a unit area is called the irradiation (or irradiance) of that area. It is given the symbol E_e and is expressed in watts per square meter. Similarly, the radiant flux emitted by a surface is called the radiant emittance, M_e, and is also expressed in watts per square meter.

If the distance between a surface and the source of the radiation is great in comparison with the size of the source, the irradiation of the surface varies inversely with the square of the distance from the source. The proportionality factor is called the radiant intensity, I_e, and is expressed in watts per steradian—that is, the power density per unit of solid angle traversing the surface.

When, as in phototherapy, the area of the radiating source is comparable with or larger than the area through which the flux is passing, the intensity per unit area becomes the important quantity. This quantity is called the radiance, is given the symbol L_e (or B), and is expressed in watts per steradian per square meter. This quantity becomes particularly important if the surface being irradiated is three-dimensional—that is, not planar. (See Appendix A.)

SPECTRORADIOMETRY

When radiation is distributed over a broad spectral region and the variation of the various radiometric quantities with wavelength is of importance, the measurement process is called spectroradiometry. The quantities measured are the same as the normal radiometric quantities; however, their names are preceded by the word *spectral,* and their symbols are subscripted by the usual symbol for wavelength, λ. The spectral quantity will depend on the width of the spectral region over which it is measured; however, as the spectral region becomes infinitesimally narrow, the amount of radiation becomes proportional to this width. We may therefore define any spectroradiometric quantity, X_λ, in terms of its radiometric counterpart, X_e, by

$$\lim_{\Delta\lambda \to 0} \frac{X_e(\lambda_0, \lambda_0 + \Delta\lambda)}{\Delta\lambda} = \frac{\partial X_e}{\partial \lambda} = X_\lambda\,(\lambda_0), \qquad (1)$$

where $\Delta\lambda$ is the width of the spectral region located at the wavelength being measured, λ_0. It should be noted that this definition of spectroradiometric quantities makes it necessary to use narrow-band detectors, if consistent and accurate results are to be obtained.

PHOTOMETRY

When a human observer is to be the detector in an optical system, knowledge of the total power emitted from a source is not enough to permit prediction of its visibility; the distribution of that power over the visible region of the spectrum must be given, and each spectral region must be weighted by a factor proportional to its effectiveness in stimulating visual response. Once this human visual response function has been established, it is possible to define photometric quantities X that are analogous to radiometric quantities X_e by

$$X = \int K(\lambda) X_e(\lambda)\, d\lambda, \tag{2}$$

where K is a function of wavelength and is the response function of the human observer. K is normally referred to as the spectral luminous efficiency.

From Table 1 we see that the photometric quantity corresponding to the radiant flux in watts is the luminous flux in lumens. The total quantity of light, Q, is given by the time integral of the luminous flux in units of lumen-seconds.

The quantities corresponding to the radiant emittance and the irradiation are the luminous emittance and the illumination; the luminous emittance is given in lumens per square meter and the illumination in lux.

The quantity corresponding to the radiant intensity is the luminous intensity and is given in candelas, while the quantity corresponding to the radiance in watts per steradian per square meter is, in luminance, given in candelas per square meter.

The examples given in Table 2 and Figure 1 are intended to give a better appreciation of the difference between radiometric and photometric measurements. In these cases, the radiometric measurement accurately quantifies the radiation from lamps used in phototherapy, but the photometric measurement does not, since much of the radiation lies in a band in which the response curve of the human eye is greatly reduced.

TABLE 2 Example of the Difference between Irradiance and Illuminance [a]

Ten 20-Watt Fluorescent Lamps	Irradiance at 425–475 nm, mW/cm^2	Illuminance, ft-c [b]
Daylight	0.3	350
Special blue	2.9	32

SOURCE: R. E. Behrman, A. K. Brown, M. R. Currie, J. W. Hastings, G. B. Odell, R. Schaffer, R. B. Setlow, T. P. Vogl, R. J. Wurtman, R. J. Anderson, H. J. Kostkowski, and A. P. Simopoulos. Preliminary report of the Committee on Phototherapy in the Newborn Infant. J. Pediatr. 84:135–143, 1974. Reprinted by permission.

[a] Specific results from a bank of ten 20-watt fluorescent lamps (daylight and special blue) placed about 18 in. from the meter.

[b] Lux in metric units.

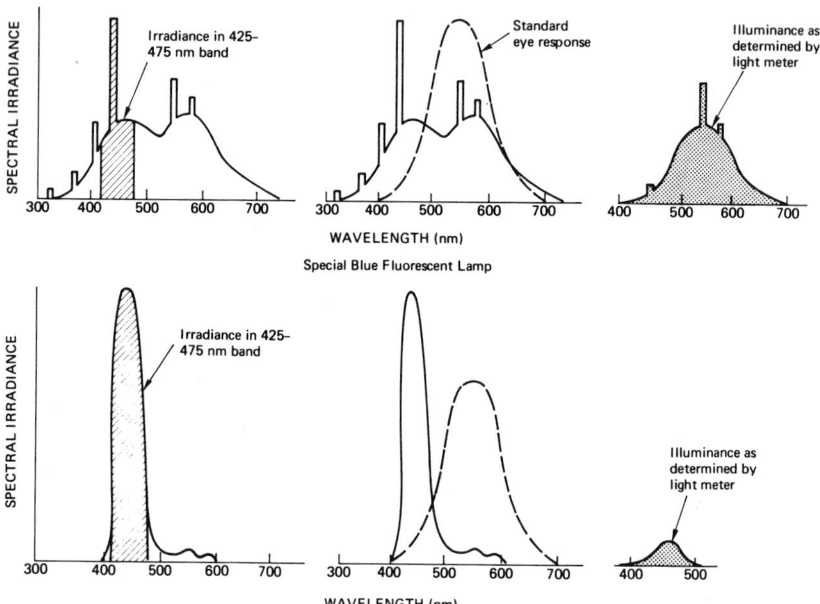

FIGURE 1 Charts illustrating the extent to which illuminance (as measured by a light meter) can differ from irradiance (as measured by a spectroradiometer) at 425–475 nm. The distributions of spectral irradiance are shown for two types of lamps commonly used for phototherapy of hyperbilirubinemia—a daylight fluorescent lamp and a special blue fluorescent lamp. Hatching shows the irradiance at 425–475 nm for each lamp, the dashed curve is the standard eye response, and the dotted area is the integral of the spectral irradiance weighted by the eye response. Irradiance at 425–475 nm is larger for the special blue lamp, but the opposite is true for illuminance. (From R. E. Behrman, A. K. Brown, M. R. Currie, J. W. Hastings, G. B. Odell, R. Schaffer, R. B. Setlow, T. P. Vogl, R. J. Wurtman, R. J. Anderson, H. J. Kostkowski, and A. P. Simopoulos. Preliminary report of the Committee on Phototherapy in the Newborn Infant. J. Pediatr. 84:135–143, 1974. Reprinted by permission.)

The derivation of a function analogous to the spectral luminous efficiency but applicable to the *in vivo* sensitivity of bilirubin to photocatabolysis is discussed in Appendix B.

The Measurement Problem in Phototherapy

Having described radiometric and photometric concepts, we now turn to the application of these concepts to the measurement problem in phototherapy. The goals of the phototherapy measurement are (1) characterization of the spectral output of the light sources used in phototherapy to document the total exposure history of the patient; (2) measurement of the irradiance impinging on the patient to ensure that a phototherapeutic dose rate is being received, particularly within the spectral region implicated in the *in vivo* photodegradation of bilirubin; and (3) measurement of the total exposure, particularly within the wavelength region implicated in the photodegradation of bilirubin, to ensure that the total light dose received is not more than is necessary to achieve the desired reduction in the level of serum bilirubin. Since, as we have seen, photometry is weighted to the visual response function of the human observer, such measurement is clearly irrelevant to the present purpose. On the other hand, while spectroradiometry can fully provide the desired information, most spectroradiometers are inappropriate for routine clinical use because they are complex and expensive. However, spectroradiometric principles can be used for the measurement and characterization of phototherapeutic dosages.

The most complex of the three goals to achieve by the measurement process as applied to phototherapy is the complete characterization of the exposure history of the patient. Difficulty arises from fluorescent lamps that emit some electromagnetic radiation in ranges outside the limits of the visible spectrum [11, 12] and often emit some relatively sharp bands. Different types of lamps have different spectral distributions over the entire region. Environmental lighting must also be considered. Thus, a complete exposure history of the patient involves the measurement, over the entire wavelength spectrum incident on the patient, of spectral irradiance expressed in W/cm^2 per unit wavelength.

One alternative to relying on the measurement of spectral irradiance at the wavelengths to which the patient is exposed would be the measurement of the power density of the incident light in relatively broad bands; such measurements would be expressed in units of W/cm^2 over the wavelength interval defined by the broadband filter. In the opinion of many photobiologists, the measurement of the power density in a number of broad bands, provided the bands were contiguous, would yield an acceptable measure of the complete exposure history of the patient. A set of contiguous bands considered useful for this purpose is indicated in Table 3.

A second alternative would require the selection of a standard lamp and standardized lamp housing material to be used for phototherapy. In principle, if the spectral output of the source and fixture can be maintained constant with time, the phototherapy source needs to be monitored only at a single wavelength to completely characterize its wavelength distribution. However, to permit this simplification, it must be

TABLE 3 Ranges for Monitoring Irradiation Exposure

Wavelength Range, nm	Reason for Consideration
Below 380	Substantially filtered out by the protective Plexiglas shields on incubators or lamps
380–425	Contains wavelengths that are absorbed by some circulating substances
425–475	The region for maximal absorption by bilirubin and many other biologic compounds, and probably implicated in the *in vivo* photochemistry of bilirubin
475–650	Contains much of the daylight spectrum important in producing the neuroendocrine effects of light
Above 650	Affects surface temperature and peripheral circulation

SOURCE: R. E. Behrman, A. K. Brown, M. R. Currie, J. W. Hastings, G. B. Odell, R. Schaffer, R. B. Setlow, T. P. Vogl, R. J. Wurtman, R. J. Anderson, H. J. Kostkowski, and A. P. Simopoulos. Preliminary report of the Committee on Phototherapy in the Newborn Infant. J. Pediatr. 84:135–143, 1974. Reprinted by permission.

emphasized that neither the lamps nor the housing can be permitted any significant change in spectral characteristics over the life of the unit.

The second goal of measurement, to ensure that the intended therapeutic dose is being administered, requires (1) that the irradiance incident on the patient within the bilirubin activation band be measured, and (2) that the total exposure, defined as the total quantity of radiation received during the entire time of the phototherapy, be recorded. In general, irradiance measurements would need to be performed only occasionally, provided that the construction of the phototherapy unit and standard operating procedures and maintenance ensure that the irradiance from the phototherapy unit remains relatively constant. Together with these periodic checks of irradiance, a set of prescribed conditions for performing phototherapy—that is, an established number of lamps placed at an established distance from the patient, in an established environment—would need to be fixed. This would suffice for the subsequent recording of the irradiance incident on the patient only if the phototherapy light source is standardized to the extent that a single type of fluorescent lamp and a single type of reflector material are used. Many kinds of reflectors, light sources, and lamp housings are used in phototherapy units at present.

The measurement of the total therapeutic exposure received during phototherapy is the last of these measurements to be considered. Assuming (1) that the light sources used in phototherapy are maintained at a constant distance from the baby during the exposure, (2) that the baby is not moved during the exposure, and (3) that the radiant flux density emitted from the lamps does not change over the duration of the exposure, it is possible to make a single measurement of the radiant flux. The product of the radiant flux and the time duration of phototherapy provides the time integral of the radiant flux, i.e., the total exposure. However, if the radiant flux is not constant over the duration of the phototherapy—for example, because the baby or the phototherapy lamp unit is moved during the exposure or because the phototherapy lamp unit is operated on an intermittent, rather than a continuous, basis—it becomes necessary to record the radiant flux effective in producing photodecomposition as a function of time and to integrate the area under this curve to obtain the radiation dose.

Radiometric Instrument for Phototherapy

Several approaches may be used in obtaining the time integral directly without the use of any mathematical processing. The first is electrical and involves the use of a detector whose output is coupled to a capacitor in such a way that the charge stored across the capacitor is proportional to the quantity of effective radiation, Q_e. (See Appendix B.) As the radiant flux increases or decreases, the incremental charge stored by the capacitor is larger or smaller; the total charge on the capacitor is proportional to Q_e.

An alternative electrical approach is to use a detector whose output is a series of pulses whose frequency is dependent upon the radiant flux detected. The total number of pulses is then counted over the duration of the phototherapy, and this number is proportional to Q_e.

A second approach, somewhat simpler than the electrical methods, is a direct optical method in which the quantity of absorbed radiation induces a proportional amount of a chemical reaction and thus measures the total quantity of chemical product formed by the radiant flux. This process, known as actinometry, is discussed in a number of textbooks on photochemistry.[5]

The special case of actinometry in which the photochemical reaction used involves a photographic emulsion is known as dosimetry [4, 16] and is used to determine the total quantity of absorbed radiation. The total light absorbed by the photographic emulsion may then simply be obtained by measuring the optical density of the emulsion in a colorimeter or densitometer and relating the measured optical density to the quantity of absorbed radiation through a suitable calibration curve. This technique is well known in the measurement of ionizing radiation.

Use of an appropriate film as a recording medium for the radiant flux makes possible the direct integration of the radiant flux for the duration of the phototherapy. With a filter matching the action spectrum of bilirubin photocatabolysis (the wavelength interval effective in phototherapy; see Appendix B) incorporated in a film badge dosimeter, the total quantity of absorbed radiation effective in phototherapy can be measured directly by its exposure in the same environment as the baby. An instrument of this type is under development by Robert J. Anderson, but none is commercially available.

Irradiance meters to cover a selected band of wavelengths (in contrast to spectroradiometers, which incorporate dispersive optical elements) are generally constructed by using photosensitive detectors preceded by a suitable spectrally selective filter. For example, interference filters can be produced by the evaporative deposition of appropriate materials of different refractive indices, each of the correct thickness (usually about one quarter wavelength). Such filters can have sharp cutoffs on both ends of the region of transparency; however, they are generally designed for use with nearly normal incident light, and if they must accept radiation over a wide distribution of angles, their spectral purity suffers unless extreme precautions are taken in their design and manufacture. Such precautions would make them prohibitively expensive for the present application. The colored glass or gelatin filters that are available can separate different portions of the visible spectrum, but these generally have sloping band pass characteristics, typically with a 150–200 nm region between the 10 percent and the 80 percent transmission points. Nonetheless, it would appear practical to produce an irradiance meter covering the bands of Table 3 by using photodiodes and colored filters.

Summary and Conclusions

In the preceding discussion we have defined the processes of radiometric and photometric measurement and have described the symbols, units, and dimensions that are appropriate to these measurement processes. Photometric instrumentation is inappropriate in the monitoring of phototherapy, since the wavelengths implicated in the *in vivo* photodecomposition of bilirubin lie well below the maximum response to instruments designed to measure visible radiation; furthermore, the fluorescent lamps used emit radiation at wavelengths both above and below the visual region. Thus, in phototherapy, the use of such instruments as photographic light meters is contraindicated.

The nature of the measurements required in clinical phototherapy has been discussed, in particular, as they apply to the three primary goals of phototherapy monitoring: (1) characterization of the spectral output of the light sources used in phototherapy, so that the total exposure history of the patient can be documented; (2) measurement of the irradiance impinging on the patient to ensure that the phototherapeutic dose rate is within the spectral region implicated in the *in vivo* photodegradation of bilirubin; and (3) measurement of the total exposure, particularly within the wavelength region implicated in the photodegradation of bilirubin, to ensure that the total light dosage received is not more than is necessary to achieve the desired reduction in the level of serum bilirubin.

The radiometric function required to ensure accurate measurement, developed in Appendix A, is extremely complex and can only be determined experimentally. It is still necessary to measure the radiant flux incident on the baby as a function of both wavelength and time and to integrate this radiant flux over wavelength and time to obtain the quantity of radiation absorbed by the baby during phototherapy. Direct measurement of the integrated quantities was found to be possible through the use of an appropriate filter/detector combination and through use of suitable time integrating devices, either electrical or chemical.

Probably the simplest means of measuring the total quantity of the absorbed radiation is the use of a photochemical actinometer, utilizing an emulsion laid down on a film base. This type of actinometer can appropriately be called a film dosimeter. The quantity of radiation absorbed by the infant during phototherapy is obtained by monitoring the optical density of the film at the conclusion of the phototherapy. The use of an appropriate filter over the film restricts the exposure of the film to the wavelength region effective in phototherapy, and the film badge dosimeter therefore integrates the radiant flux over both wavelength and time.

Although neither suitable irradiance measuring instruments nor dosimeters for measuring total exposure received during phototherapy are commercially available, it is apparent that the continued use of phototherapy will make it necessary to produce these instruments commercially. It should be realized, however, that biochemical research is still required to elucidate the action spectrum *in vivo,* and this knowledge is essential for construction of an appropriate filter.

APPENDIX A: CALCULATING THE LIGHT INCIDENT ON A BABY UNDER PHOTOTHERAPY

Total Light

We simplify the calculation of the total light received by a baby under phototherapy by assuming that the baby can be represented by a cylinder whose diameter equals the chest diameter of the baby. We further assume that the cylinder is infinitely long and therefore can compute the total light incident per unit length on the baby. The cross-sectional geometry is shown in Figure 2.

The light received by the circle representing the baby from any point on the lamp is

$$B \int_{\phi_0}^{\phi_1} \cos\phi \, d\phi, \tag{1}$$

where B is a constant determined by the radiance of the lamp and ϕ is an angle measured from the normal, N, to the lamp, of halfwidth L, which varies between the angles ϕ_0 and ϕ_1. The included angle subtends the infant.

The total direct light (TDL) is the sum of light from each point on the lamp:

$$\text{TDL} = \int_{-L}^{L} \int_{\phi_0}^{\phi_1} B \cos\phi \, d\phi \, d\ell. \tag{2}$$

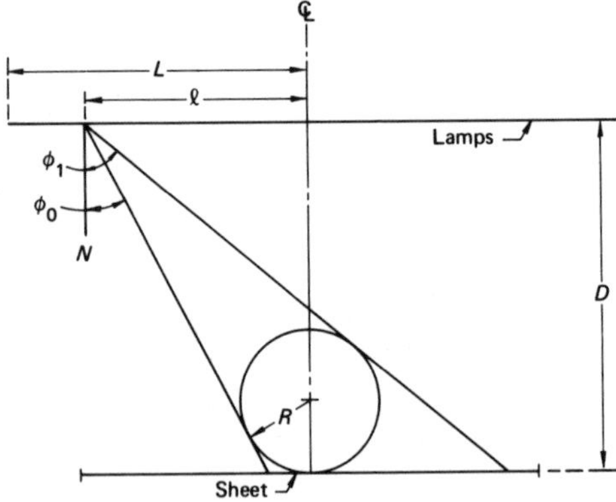

FIGURE 2 Cross-sectional representation of a baby on a sheet under a bank of lamps. R is the radius of the baby (measured at the sternum), D is the separation of the sheet from the lights, L is the semiwidth of the lamp bank, ℓ is an arbitrary point within L, N is a normal drawn to the lamp bank, and ϕ_0 and ϕ_1 are the angles from point ℓ that are tangent to the baby.

The value of this integral is

$$\text{TDL} = 4\ BR \arctan\ (L/(D-R)). \quad (3)$$

Note that if the lamp is curved or segmented, the calculations are performed for an equivalent flat lamp as illustrated in Figure 3. It is, therefore, a limitation of the present calculation method that the lowest point on the lamp must be higher than the highest point on the infant.

To determine the light reflected from the sheet, we need to calculate the light received by each point on the sheet. The power received at the sheet from the lamp is diffused by the sheet. Let $B(y)$ be the effective radiance of a point on the sheet at a distance y (Figure 4) from the intersection of the baby from the sheet. Then the emitted irradiance is

$$E_{\text{emitted}} = \int_{-\pi/2}^{\pi/2} B(y) \cos\phi \, d\phi = 2B(y). \quad (4)$$

In the above, the angle ϕ is measured from the normal to the point on the sheet. Since the emitted irradiance equals the received irradiance multiplied by the reflectivity μ of the sheet,

$$B(y) = \mu/2\ x, \quad (5)$$

where x is the received irradiance.

The irradiance received on a point y on the sheet is B multiplied by the integral of the cosine of the angle that a ray of light makes with the normal to the sheet as the ray varies along the width of the lamp or perhaps until it is blocked by the shadow of the baby.

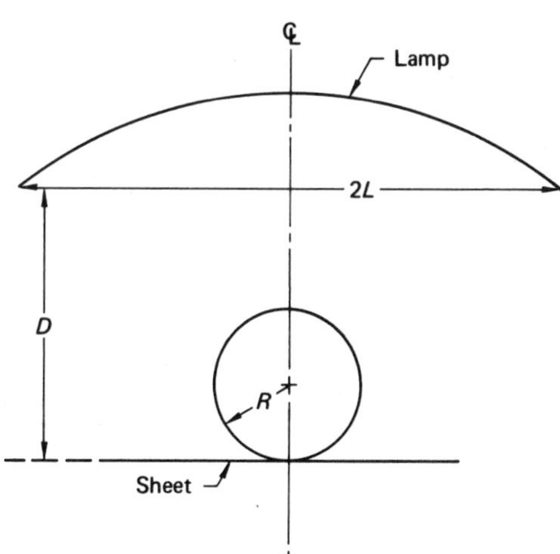

FIGURE 3 Cross-sectional representation of a baby on a sheet under a curved lamp bank. A curved lamp bank can be evaluated on the same basis as a flat bank of equal brightness, provided that the distances L and D are measured as shown.

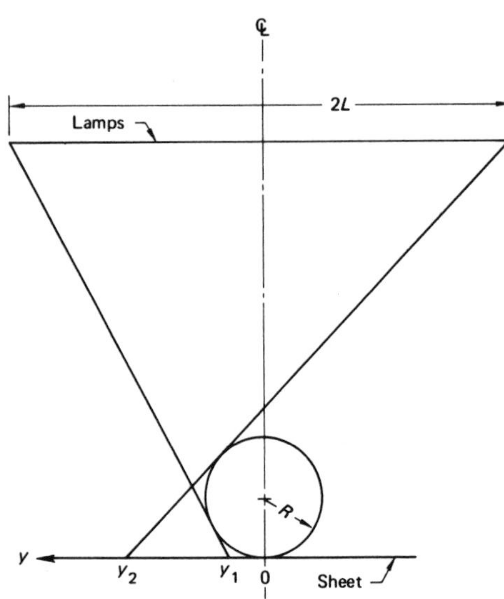

FIGURE 4 Cross-sectional representation for calculation of partial shading for a baby on a sheet under a bank of lamps. The region on the sheet directly under the baby, from 0 to y_1, is completely shaded by the baby. The region between y_1 and y_2 receives only part of the direct light and is therefore partly in shade. The region beyond y_2 is in full light. This figure illustrates the derivation of the reflected light from the sheet falling on the baby.

If $y > y_2$, the baby causes no shadowing. It can be determined that

$$B(y) = \frac{\mu B}{2}\left[\frac{L+y}{\sqrt{D^2+(L+y)^2}} + \frac{L-y}{\sqrt{D^2+(L-y)^2}}\right]. \qquad (6)$$

If $y_1 < y < y_2$,

$$B(y) = \frac{\mu B}{2}\left[\frac{L-y}{\sqrt{D^2+(L-y)^2}} + \frac{y^2-R^2}{y^2+R^2}\right]. \qquad (7)$$

If $y < y_1$, no light reaches the sheet and $B(y) = 0$.

The light reflected to the baby from a point y on the sheet is the radiance of that point multiplied by the integral of the cosine of the angle that a light ray makes with the normal to the sheet over the angle subtended by the baby. This may be evaluated as

$$2B(y)\ R^2/(R^2+y^2). \qquad (8)$$

Thus, the total reflected light (TRL) on the baby is

$$\text{TRL} = 2R^2 \int_{-y_3}^{y_3} \frac{B(y)}{y^2+R^2}\, dy, \qquad (9)$$

where y_3 is the semiwidth of the bed. We can now insert the appropriate values of $B(y)$ and obtain

$$\mathrm{TRL} = 2\mu BR^2 \left\{ \int_{y_1}^{y_3} \frac{(L-y)}{(y^2+R^2)\sqrt{D^2+(L-y)^2}}\, dy + \int_{y_1}^{y_2} \frac{y^2-R^2}{(y^2+R^2)^2}\, dy + \int_{y_2}^{y_3} \frac{(L+y)}{(y^2+R^2)\sqrt{D^2+(L+y)^2}}\, dy \right\} \quad (10)$$

The results of evaluating this function are plotted in Figure 5 for a typical commercial Bililight 48 cm deep located 70 cm above a bed 36 cm wide. The irradiance at the sternum is assumed to be 1 μW/cm^2 so that the results plotted are in units of μW/cm of the baby's length per μW/cm^2 incident on the sternum. We have assumed that the reflectivity of the sheet is 0.75. We observe that the reflected irradiance is nearly constant over the range of common infant circumferences and the total and direct irradiances are practically linear functions of circumference.

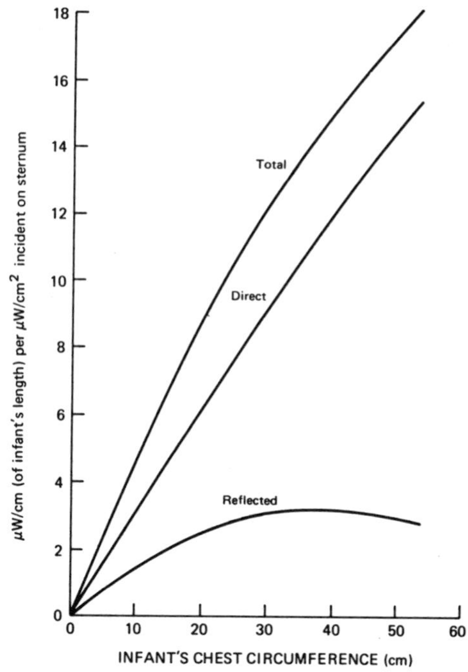

FIGURE 5 Components of the total optical power incident on the baby. The total power incident on the baby per unit of its length may be found from these curves. To find the power incident on the baby due to direct light from the lamps, or to reflected light from the sheet, or to their sum (the total light), multiply the value in μW/cm per μW/cm^2 obtained for the infant's chest circumference by the irradiance measured at the sternum. This will yield the power incident per unit length of the baby. Multiplying this number by the length of the baby will give the total radiant flux in watts. Here and in Figure 7, a sheet reflectivity of 0.75, light depth $L = 48$ cm, and a bed width $2y_3 = 36$ cm have been assumed.

Irradiance at a Point on the Baby

We shall now calculate the irradiance received at any point P on the baby as a function of the angle θ illustrated in Figure 6.

As before, the direct irradiance at P is found by multiplying B by the integral of the cosine of the angle that a ray of light from the lamp makes with the normal at P. The limits of this integral are determined by the tangent line to the circle at P. Let y_0 be the intersection of this line with the sheet.

If $y_0 \geq y_2$, P receives light from the entire lamp. By evaluating the integral described above, we find the direct irradiance $E_d(\theta)$ to be

$$E_d(\theta)=B\left[\frac{(D-R)\sin\theta+L\cos\theta}{\sqrt{(L+R\sin\theta)^2+(D-R-R\cos\theta)^2}}+\frac{L\cos\theta-(D-R)\sin\theta}{\sqrt{(L-R\sin\theta)^2+(D-R-R\cos\theta)^2}}\right]. \quad (11)$$

If $y_1 < y_0 < y_2$, only part of the lamp illuminates P and

$$E_d(\theta)=B\left[1+\frac{L\cos\theta-(D-R)\sin\theta}{\sqrt{(L-R\sin\theta)^2+(D-R-P\cos\theta)^2}}\right]. \quad (12)$$

If $y_0 \leq y_1$, no direct light reaches P; that is, $E_d(\theta)=0$.

The position of the tangent line at P also determines the reflected light $E_r(\theta)$ reaching P. If y_0 extends past the edge of the bed defined

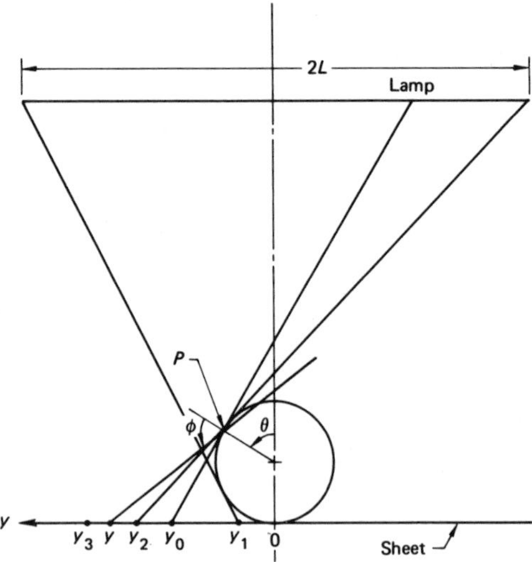

FIGURE 6 Cross-sectional representation for evaluation of the light at a point on the circumference of a baby on a sheet under a bank of lamps. The line tangent to the circle at P intersects the plane of the sheet at y_0 and intersects the lamp so as to divide it into two portions. One of the portions contributes direct light at P and the other does not. Light is reflected onto P from point y on the sheet between y_0 to y_3; y_3 is the edge of the bed.

by the point y_3, then no reflected light is incident at P and $E_r(\theta) = 0$. If $y_0 < y_3$,

$$E_r(\theta) = \int_{\phi(y_3)}^{\phi(y_0)} B(\phi) \cos \phi \, d\phi, \qquad (13)$$

where ϕ is the angle that a reflected ray of light with radiance $B(\phi)$ makes with the normal to the circle at P. This integral may be expressed in terms of y instead of ϕ:

$$E_r(\theta) = \int_{y_0}^{y_3} B(y) \frac{[y \sin \theta - R(1+\cos \theta)]}{[R^2(1+\cos \theta)^2 + (y - R \sin \theta)^2]^{3/2}} dy, \qquad (14)$$

where $B(y)$ vanishes or is given by Eq. (6) or Eq. (7), depending on the value of y.

Equation (14) can be integrated directly by numerical methods or it can be expressed in closed form in terms of elliptic integrals, which we will omit for the sake of simplicity.

The total irradiance at P is found by adding $E_d(\theta)$ to $E_r(\theta)$. The variation of irradiance along the circumference of several typical infants is shown in Figure 7 for the same bed and light characteristics as given in the previous section. In this figure the energy per square centimeter

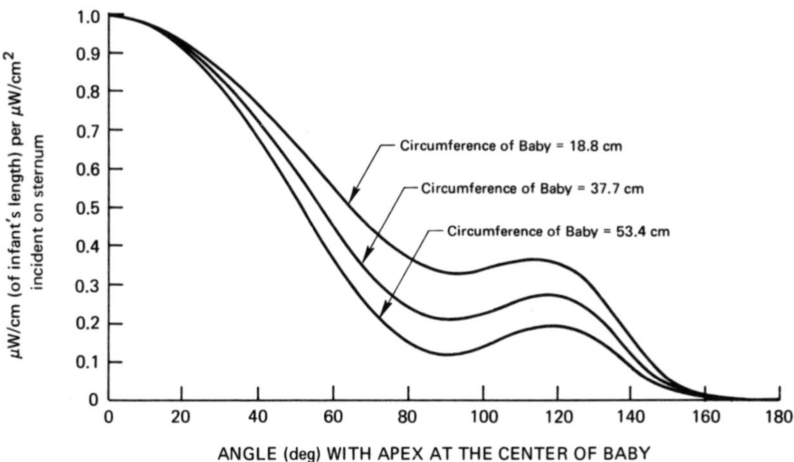

FIGURE 7 Normalized irradiance on circumference of baby. To find the irradiance at a point on the circumference of the baby given by the angle θ (defined in Figure 6), where 0° represents the baby's sternum, multiply the ordinate of the point appropriate for that angle and the baby's circumference by the irradiance measured at the sternum.

incident on the surface of the baby is plotted against the angle on the baby at which that power is incident. To obtain the total power per linear centimeter of the baby from this curve, the area under the curve must be multiplied by the circumference of the baby and divided by 360 (to convert degrees into 2π radians).

The equations given and the sample curves of Figures 5 and 7 permit one to calculate the irradiance incident on a baby from a large class of phototherapy units both in terms of the irradiance per unit length of the infant and in terms of the angular dependence of the irradiance around the circumference of the baby. Persons interested in obtaining copies of the computer program are invited to write directly to the third author.

APPENDIX B: DETERMINATION OF THE *IN VIVO* ACTION SPECTRUM OF BILIRUBIN

The work of Cremer *et al.*,[6] Hewitt *et al.*,[7] Ostrow and Branham,[15] and others, as well as consideration of the photochemical process, leads to the conclusion that some wavelengths of light are more effective in decomposing bilirubin than others. It follows, even though we do not know its exact shape, that a curve of *in vivo* effectiveness in bilirubin decomposition versus wavelength must exist. The ordinate of such a curve would be in units of molecules of bilirubin decomposed per photon or per watt of absorbed energy in a certain wavelength interval. (Note that the word *absorbed* is used; light that is not absorbed cannot participate in the photochemical process.) Such a curve could also be viewed as a curve of quantum efficiency of bilirubin photodegradation versus wavelength. Conceptually, it is equivalent to the spectral luminous efficiency (see p. 5), which is proportional to the quantum efficiency of the eye.

Attempts to derive the shape of this curve theoretically on the basis of chemical kinetics quickly lead to mathematically intractable formulations. Not only is the order of the reaction unknown, but the rate-limiting step (which may not be the photochemical step) and its kinetics are also unknown. The problem is compounded further by the fact that, as the light decomposes the bilirubin, more bilirubin is being generated by the infant. Another difficulty is that the light, instead of interacting with the bilirubin in the vascular space, may interact in the cutaneous and subcutaneous tissue.[10] Before a meaningful theoretical model can be built, we must take into account the diffusion dynamics of the bilirubin into that space, how easily it diffuses back out as the serum bilirubin level drops, and how easily the degradation products diffuse out. All this is the appropriate subject for research that should be undertaken as soon as possible.

An alternative approach would be to determine the *in vivo* action spectrum clinically. Groups of infants could be irradiated with narrow bands of radiation and the effect on serum bilirubin determined. If the bands are sufficiently narrow and span the range of effective wavelengths, the action spectrum *in vivo* would be established. However, it must be borne in mind that in each band the effect of the light will probably depend on the spectral irradiance (that is, the effect may not be linear with spectral irradiance) and that, in addition, the effect may depend on the degree of jaundice as well as the length of time the patient has been jaundiced and the amount of cutaneous and subcutaneous tissue and the effectiveness of peripheral circulation. Thus, the experiment is not easy to perform. However, even a simple experiment of this kind conducted on a group of "typically" jaundiced infants could give a good initial estimate of the action spectrum.

Once the action spectrum *in vivo* has been determined, even approximately, it is possible to construct either a dosimeter or an irradiance meter that will faithfully measure the therapeutic dose or dose rate. It would consist of a photosensitive element, chemical or electronic, whose spectral response is known. A filter could then be constructed with a spectral transmission chosen in such a way that the product of its transmission curve and the spectral response curve of the sensing device is the same as the action spectrum for photodegradation of bilirubin.

Ultimately, such a device would be ideal for the clinical monitoring of the phototherapeutic dose.

REFERENCES

1. American National Standards Institute. Rules for the Use of Units of the International System of Units and a Selection of the Decimal Multiples and Sub-Multiples of the SI Units. New York: American National Standards Institute, 1969.
2. American Society for Testing and Materials. ASTM Standard Metric Practice Guide. A Guide to the Use of SI—The International Systems of Units. Designation: E–380–70. Philadelphia: American Society for Testing and Materials, 1970.
3. American Standards Association. ASA Standard Z7.1. Illuminating Engineering Nomenclature and Photometric Standards. New York: American Standards Association.
4. Brown, G. H., Ed. Photochromism. Techniques of Chemistry. Vol. 3. New York: John Wiley & Sons, Inc., 1971. 853 pp.
5. Calvert, J. G., and J. N. Pitts, Jr. Experimental methods in photochemistry,

pp. 686–814. In J. G. Calvert and J. N. Pitts, Jr., Eds. Photochemistry. New York: John Wiley & Sons, Inc., 1966.

6. Cremer, R. J., P. W. Perryman, and D. H. Richards. Influence of light on the hyperbilirubinaemia of infants. Lancet 1:1094–1097, 1958.
7. Hewitt, J. R., R. M. Klein, and J. F. Lucey. Photodegradation of serum bilirubin in the Gunn rat. Biol. Neonate 21:112–119, 1972.
8. IEEE recommended practice for units in published scientific and technical work. I.E.E.E. Spectrum 3(3):169–173, 1966.
9. International Union of Pure and Applied Physics. Symbols, units and nomenclature on physics. Physics Today 15:20–30, 1962. Compare also the 1965 Revision: UIP–11, SUN65–3.
10. Kapoor, C. L., C. R. Krishna Murti, and P. C. Bajpai. Uptake and release of bilirubin by skin. Biochem. J. 136:35–43, 1973.
11. Kaufman, J. E., and J. F. Christensen, Eds. IES Lighting Handbook. (5th ed.) New York: Illuminating Engineering Society, 1972.
12. Levi, L. Applied Optics; A Guide to Optical System Design. New York: John Wiley & Sons, Inc., 1968. 620 pp.
13. Mechtly, E. A. The International System of Units—Physical Constants and Conversion Factors. (2nd Rev. ed.) NASA Publication No. SP–7012. Washington, D.C.: U.S. Government Printing Office, 1973. 21 pp.
14. Moon, P. H. The Scientific Basis of Illuminating Engineering. (Rev. ed.) New York: Dover Publications, Inc., 1961. 608 pp.
15. Ostrow, J. D., and R. V. Branham. Photodecomposition of bilirubin and biliverdin *in vitro*. Gastroenterology 58:15–25, 1970.
16. Price, W. J. Nuclear Radiation Detection, pp. 211–254. New York: McGraw-Hill Book Co., 1958.

CHRISTOPHER S. FOOTE

Photooxidation

Organic molecules on absorption of light are converted to chemically reactive electronically excited states. Only light that is absorbed can cause photochemical reactions. Absorption of light promotes an electron to a higher orbital without change of spin; thus, the first state formed is the singlet, in which there are no unpaired spins.

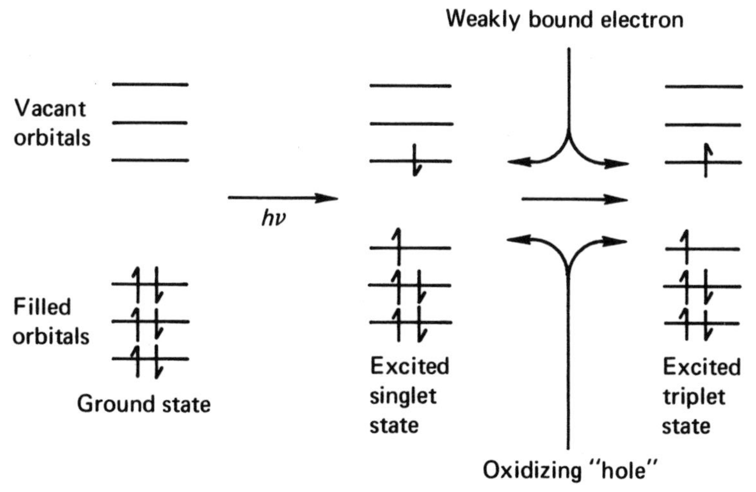

There are many mechanisms of photooxidation, but only those that take place in the presence of oxygen are discussed here.

The singlet in many cases undergoes a spin inversion very rapidly to give the triplet state (which has two unpaired electrons). Usually the triplet state lasts much longer than the singlet; both states involve electrons promoted to higher orbitals. As these orbitals bind the electrons less strongly than do those of the ground state, one would expect that electrons in these orbitals would be more readily removed by oxidizing agents than would those in the ground state. By the same token, the holes left by the promoted electron are in orbitals that bind electrons comparatively strongly; thus, one would expect that the excited molecule that results would be more readily susceptible to reducing agents than would the molecule in the ground state. Both expectations are realized: Excited singlet and triplet molecules are both oxidized and reduced more readily than ground-state molecules; oxidizing behavior is especially common.

Photosensitized oxygenations of organic compounds have been studied for many years.[17, 18, 25] The interest of chemists was attracted by biologists' observation that the combination of sensitizing dyes, light, and oxygen is capable of damaging organisms of virtually all classes.[39, 41–43] The effects (referred to as *photodynamic action*) include membrane damage, mutagenesis, interference with metabolism, and death. The chemical basis of these effects has been traced to damage to many different cell constituents, including lipids (which are peroxidized) and certain enzymes and peptides (methionine, histidine, tryptophane, and tyrosine are the most susceptible to photosensitized oxidation), and to nucleic acids (the guanine residues are the most sensitive).[39, 41–43] Recent studies have led to greatly increased understanding in this area. It is now possible to recognize several distinct mechanistic pathways, and to make a beginning in predicting which mechanism will occur in a given case.[9]

With few exceptions, sensitized oxidations proceed via the sensitizer triplet state, at least in part because the lifetime of the triplet is much longer than that of the singlet.[9, 17, 18, 25, 39, 41–43] The most effective sensi-

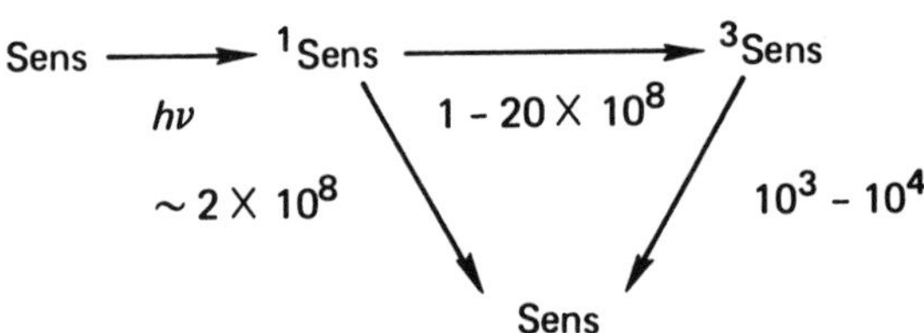

FIGURE 1 Diagram showing rates per second of internal electronic processes for typical photosensitizing dyes.

tizers are those that give a long-lived triplet state with high quantum yield. Many dyes, such as methylene blue or eosin, natural pigments (chlorophyll, hematoporphyrin, flavins), and aromatic hydrocarbons (rubrene, anthracene), are effective sensitizers. Bilirubin appears to be a weak sensitizer. Most of these compounds absorb visible or long ultraviolet light, the effective wavelengths for photodynamic action. Figure 1 shows rates of formation and deactivation of the two excited states of typical sensitizing dyes.[17]

Mechanistic Classification

There are two broad classes of reaction open to the sensitizer triplet.[36] The first is one in which the sensitizer interacts with another molecule directly, usually with a hydrogen atom or electron transfer. The radicals thus formed undergo further reaction with oxygen or other organic molecules. This reaction has been classed Type I by Gollnick.[17] The second class of reaction, Type II, is one in which the sensitizer triplet interacts with oxygen. The most common of the Type II interactions has been shown to be energy transfer to give singlet molecular oxygen, which reacts further with various acceptors in solution.[10, 21] Less efficiently, electron transfer to oxygen occurs with the formation of the superoxide ion ($O_2^{\cdot -}$); this reaction occurs in less than 1 percent of the deactivating collisions of oxygen with the sensitizer triplet.[20, 22] These reactions are summarized in Figure 2.

The rates of reaction, k_{I} and k_{II}, of the two processes are now well enough known that many of the factors governing them can be stated definitively. The rate of the Type I process depends on the sensitizer and the substrate and varies over a wide range. Table 1 shows how this

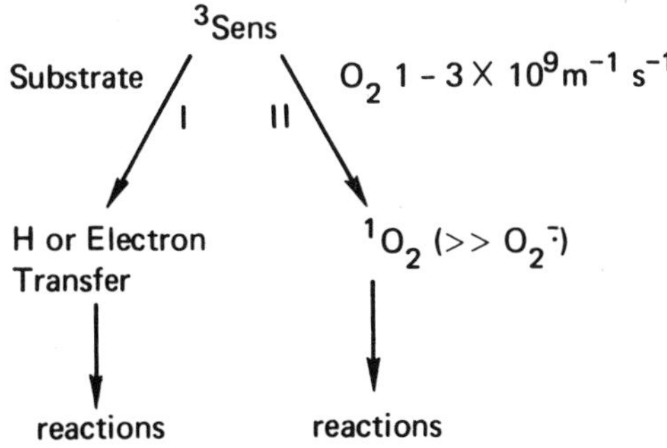

FIGURE 2 Diagram of processes involving the sensitizer triplet.

TABLE 1 Rates of Type I Process

Solvent	Rates of Reaction (k_I) with Sensitizer, $M^{-1}s^{-1}$	
	Benzophenone	Eosin
Ethanol	$\sim 10^6$ [a]	~ 100 [b]
Dimethylaniline [c]	2.7×10^9 [d]	2×10^9 [e]

[a] Rate for isopropyl alcohol. Data from Sherman and Cohen.[37]
[b] Data from Nemoto *et al.*[32]
[c] Quenching + reaction.
[d] Data from Cohen and Litt.[7]
[e] Data from C. S. Foote and R. Denny, unpublished.

rate varies for a few selected cases. It is seen that benzophenone is a stronger hydrogen abstracter than eosin toward ethanol, by a factor of 4 powers of ten. Both benzophenone and eosin are capable of reacting very rapidly, however, toward the much stronger reductant dimethylaniline. In general, as might be expected, the types of molecular structure that favor Type I (substrate-sensitizer) chemistry are those that are readily oxidized (phenols, amines, etc.) or readily reduced (quinones, etc.). Compounds that are not so readily oxidized or reduced (olefins, dienes, aromatic compounds) more often favor Type II reactions; however, Type II reactions of amines,[38] phenols,[34] and other substrates are also known. The rates for the Type II process depend mainly on the oxygen concentration in solution, since the rate constant (k_{II}) with few exceptions falls in the range $1-3 \times 10^9$ $M^{-1}s^{-1}$ for all sensitizers.[17, 44] Thus, for example, oxygen is much less soluble in water than in most organic solvents, so that in studies carried out in water saturated with air, the product k_{II} $[O_2]$ is much smaller than in organic solvents saturated with oxygen, as shown in Table 2. Unfortunately, biologists have tended to favor studies under the former set of conditions,

TABLE 2 Rates of Type II Process [a]

Condition	$k_{II}[O_2]$, s^{-1}	Reference
Water saturated with air	$\sim 5 \times 10^5$	A. McDonagh, p. 56, this volume
Organic solvents saturated with oxygen	$\sim 2 \times 10^7$	Ref. 16

[a] Assuming $k_{II} \sim 2 \times 10^9$ $M^{-1}s^{-1}$.

whereas most mechanistic chemical studies have been carried out under the latter.

The significant competition that determines whether Type I or Type II reaction occurs is thus between substrate and oxygen for triplet sensitizer. Table 3 shows that, for benzophenone in oxygen-saturated ethanol, the Type I process (with solvent ethanol) competes effectively with the Type II process; however, with eosin under the same conditions, the Type II process predominates and would continue to predominate even at very low oxygen concentration. It is probable that the same is true for bilirubin. Thus, changes in sensitizer, substrate, or concentrations of substrate and oxygen may change the mechanism of the photooxidation from Type I to Type II. It is also important to recognize that binding of dye to macromolecular substrates is likely to favor Type I mechanisms.[5, 45]

Products of the Reaction

Type I chemistry usually involves the production of free radicals or radical ions. These radicals have a very wide variety of possible reactions, such as reaction with or electron transfer to oxygen, electron or hydrogen abstraction from other substrates, initiation of chain autoxidation, and recombination. Many apparently simple reactions of this type are found to involve complex sequences of reactions when scrutinized carefully. For example, the oxidized dye formed by electron donation to oxygen or another oxidizing species (including another dye molecule) can oxidize the substrate, regenerating dye and giving a new reactive species capable of further reaction or recombination with reduced primary oxidant (Figure 3).[20, 22]

If the end fate is recombination, there may be no visible reaction, and only by probing with such techniques as flash spectroscopy or chemical trapping can the intermediacy of these species be detected. There are many similar types of complex reaction involving electron transfer to or

TABLE 3 Competitive Rates of Type I and Type II Processes for Triplet-State Sensitizer in Ethanol

Sensitizer	Rates of Reaction by Type, s^{-1}	
	$k_I[S]$	$k_{II}[O_2]$
$(C_6H_5)_2C{=}0$	$\sim 10^7$	$\sim 2 \times 10^7$
Eosin	$\sim 10^3$	$\sim 2 \times 10^7$

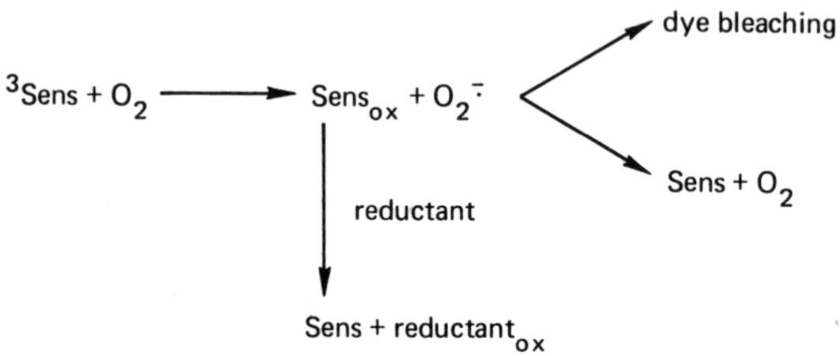

FIGURE 3 Diagram of interaction of the sensitizer triplet with oxidizing substrates.

from excited dye and substrate or the dye itself. Koizumi has subclassified Type I reactions as D–D (interaction with dye) and D–R (interaction with substrate) and refers to Type II reactions as D–O (interaction with oxygen).[23] Another example of a complex reaction is given in Figure 4.[32] Figure 5 gives two examples of Type I reactions: the oxidation of alcohols by benzophenone, which can lead either to ketone or hydroxyhydroperoxide, depending on the conditions,[35] and the oxidation of amines, which may proceed either by hydrogen or electron transfer.[3]

The Type II reaction produces singlet molecular oxygen as the primary reactive species.[10, 21] There are two excited states of singlet oxygen. The higher, $^1\Sigma_g^+$, has an energy of 37 kcal; its lifetime in solution is believed not to exceed 10^{-11} s. The lower energy state, $^1\Delta_g$, lasts much longer and is now believed to be the only singlet oxygen species that is reactive. The higher $^1\Sigma_g^+$ state, if it is formed at all, appears to be quenched to the $^1\Delta_g$ state before reacting. The lifetime of $^1\Delta_g$ oxygen has recently been determined by direct methods and is moderately subject to influence by solvent. The lifetime is shortest in hydroxylic solvents: In water, the lifetime is about 10^{-6} s.[1, 15, 29, 30] In aprotic solvents, and particularly in those with no hydrogens whatever, the lifetime is longer and reaches several hundred microseconds.

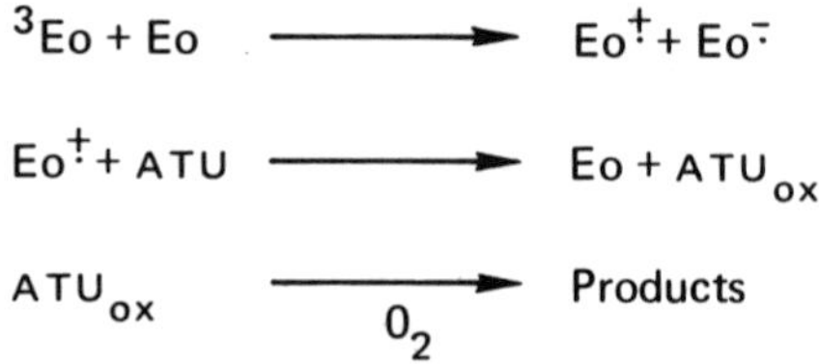

FIGURE 4 Diagram of D–D oxidation of allylthiourea (ATU). Eo = eosin.

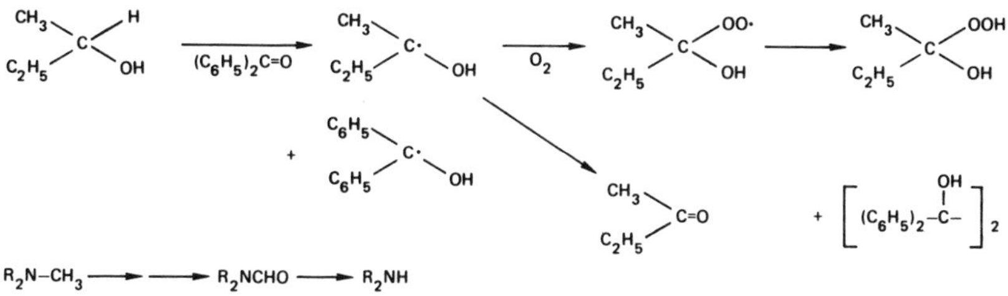

$$CH_3(C_2H_5)C(H)OH \xrightarrow{(C_6H_5)_2C=O} CH_3(C_2H_5)\dot{C}OH + (C_6H_5)_2\dot{C}OH$$

$$CH_3(C_2H_5)\dot{C}OH \xrightarrow{O_2} CH_3(C_2H_5)C(OO\cdot)OH \longrightarrow CH_3(C_2H_5)C(OOH)OH$$

$$CH_3(C_2H_5)\dot{C}OH \longrightarrow CH_3(C_2H_5)C=O + [(C_6H_5)_2C(OH)-]_2$$

$$R_2N-CH_3 \longrightarrow \longrightarrow R_2NCHO \longrightarrow R_2NH$$

FIGURE 5 Examples of Type I reactions.

TABLE 4 Rates of Reaction of Some Typical Substrates with $^1O_2$

Acceptor	k_A, $M^{-1}s^{-1}$
2,5-Dimethylfuran	1.4×10^8
2,3-Dimethyl-2-butene	5×10^7
2-Methyl-2-pentene	1×10^6
1-Methylcyclohexene	2×10^5
Cyclohexene	3×10^3
trans-4-Methyl-2-pentene	3×10^3

SOURCE: Foote,[10] Adams and Wilkinson,[1] Merkel and Kearns,[29] Merkel *et al.*,[30] and Foote *et al.*[15]

There is thus a second competition, between the decay rate of singlet oxygen and the product $k_A[A]$; if $k_A[A] << k_d$, the main result of a Type II reaction is simply the quenching of triplet sensitizer, and again one may observe no reaction at all. Rates for some typical substrates are given in Table 4. The rate for bilirubin has not been determined but is probably very large.*

Certain dyes that are less efficient oxidizers can also transfer an electron to oxygen, giving an oxidized dye molecule and superoxide ion.[20, 22] For example, eosin reduces oxygen on a small fraction (<1%) of quenching collisions;[20, 22] the other collisions give singlet oxy-

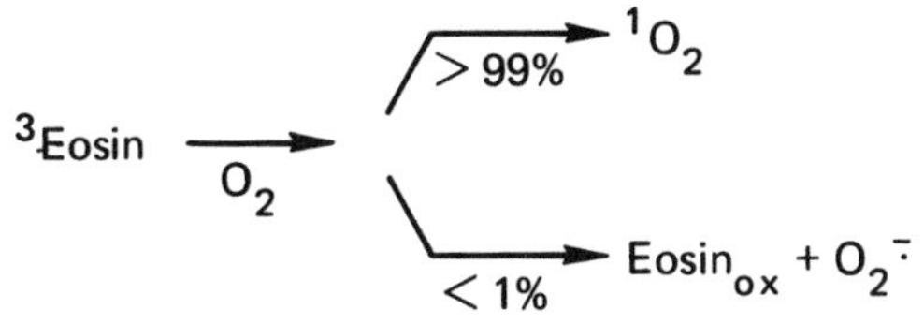

$$^3\text{Eosin} \xrightarrow{O_2} \begin{cases} \xrightarrow{>99\%} {}^1O_2 \\ \xrightarrow{<1\%} \text{Eosin}_{ox} + O_2^{\overline{\cdot}} \end{cases}$$

* We have recently determined the rate of reaction of bilirubin with singlet oxygen to be 2.5×10^9 $M^{-1}s^{-1}$, the remainder being physical quenching (C. S. Foote and T.-Y. Ching, in preparation).

gen.[10,17,18,21,25] The subsequent chemistry of the oxidized dye and superoxide is not well established. In some cases, the oxidized dye appears to oxidize the substrate (for example, trytophane or tyrosine);[20,22] however, the overall efficiency of this path (which may be one of the major causes of dye bleaching) is low, and a singlet oxygen mechanism for the main path of tryptophane and tyrosine oxidation has not been ruled out. The chemistry of $O_2^{\cdot -}$ is largely that of electron transfer to reducible substrates (for example, cytochrome, tetrazolium blue).[2,28,31]

Two classes of reaction of singlet oxygen are particularly important: addition to olefins, giving allylic hydroperoxides, analogous to the Alder "ene" reaction of Eq. (1), and additions to diene systems to produce endoperoxides, analogous to the Diels–Alder reaction of Eq. (2).[9,17,18,25,36]

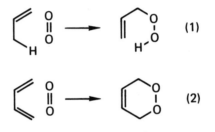

(1)

(2)

To these should be added two other classes of somewhat less generality, a 2+2 cycloaddition to electron-rich olefins (e.g., enamines and vinyl ethers) and a very few other olefins to produce dioxetanes [Eq. (3)], which are sometimes of moderate stability but readily cleave into two carbonyl-containing fragments,[4,13,27] and oxidation of certain heteroatoms, notably sulfur and phosphorus [Eq. (4)], a reaction exemplified by the oxidation of diethyl sulfide to diethyl sulfoxide, in which two moles of sulfoxide are formed for each mole of oxygen consumed.[14] Oxidation of bilirubin appears to combine reactions of the second and third classes. The intermediacy of singlet oxygen has been shown

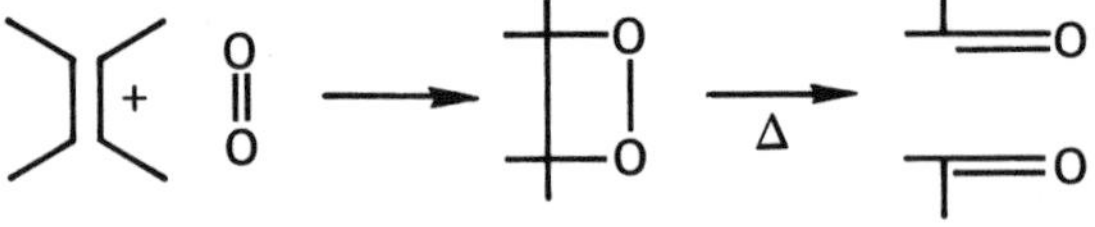

(3)

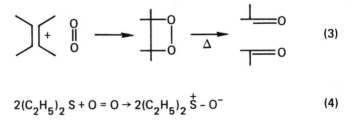

$$2(C_2H_5)_2S + O{=}O \rightarrow 2(C_2H_5)_2\overset{+}{S}{-}O^- \qquad (4)$$

rigorously for each of these reactions by careful mechanistic studies.[4, 8, 10, 13, 14, 21, 27] Under ordinary conditions (dye sensitizer, oxygen-saturated in organic solvent, dilute substrate), Type I mechanisms do not occur for these types of substrate. Certain phenols and amines have also been shown to react with singlet oxygen; these reactions may well involve hydrogen or electron abstraction by singlet oxygen, and the overall chemistry resembles that observed in Type I cases.[34, 38] Amines and phenols can also quench singlet oxygen; the mechanism of this quenching may also involve electron transfer.[34, 38] These reactions, however, will require a great deal more study before their nature is thoroughly understood.

One other significant interaction with oxygen has been established. One of the functions of carotenes in photosynthetic organisms appears to be protection against photodynamic damage to the organism by various natural sensitizers.[24] For example, carotenoidless mutants or plants in which carotene synthesis is blocked are known to be killed by light and oxygen under conditions that are normally harmless. Carotenoids have also been shown to protect organisms against exogenous sensitizers. Carotenes are known to quench triplet dyes at a very high rate, but we have also shown that they are extremely efficient quenchers of singlet oxygen.[12] Furthermore, the efficiency of quenching is a function of the number of conjugated double bonds in the polyene chain; those carotenes with nine or more conjugated double bonds are efficient quenchers, whereas those with seven or fewer quench only inefficiently or not at all.[11] This is also the range in which the effectiveness of natural carotenes in protection of organisms changes; those with nine or more double bonds are effective protective agents, whereas those with eight or fewer are less effective or ineffective.[24, 26] This parallelism suggests that quenching of singlet oxygen may be an important mechanism of protection against the photodynamic effect and that singlet oxygen is important in at least some types of photodynamic effect.[11]

The various reactions that have been shown to occur with triplet sensitizers are shown in Figure 6; careful study of this figure shows how sensitive the course of the reaction can be to conditions. Several authors have demonstrated the switch from one mechanism to another by simply changing conditions.[6, 40]

Several methods for distinguishing Type I and Type II mechanisms are now available. Simple kinetic studies may be misleading since both Type I and Type II reactions can give Stern–Volmer plots under the right conditions. One of the most powerful techniques for demonstrating the intermediacy of singlet oxygen is by competitive inhibition with a known singlet oxygen acceptor that is not a good Type I substrate.[9, 19] Very few such substrates are known that are soluble in water, however;

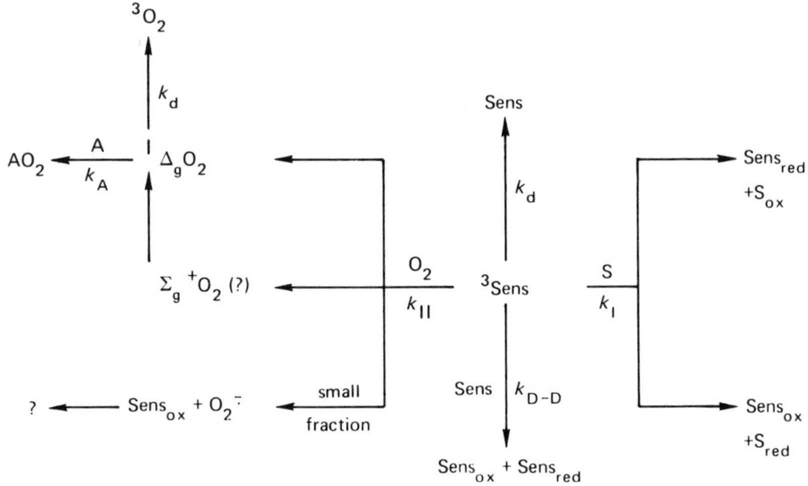

FIGURE 6 Summary of reactions with triplet sensitizers.

we are now studying some water-soluble carotenoids and olefins that may be satisfactory substrates.

Kearns has recently developed a technique for demonstrating singlet oxygen intermediacy based on the fact that the lifetime of singlet oxygen is much longer in D_2O than in H_2O; this may give a higher rate of reaction in D_2O than in water.[33] However, there are assumptions that must be made before this technique can be used. The assumption that there is no change in efficiency of the Type I reaction in D_2O as compared with H_2O has not yet been tested. Also, this technique will yield positive results only if the singlet oxygen reaction is in the first order range—that is, where $k_A[A] < k_d$; if the reverse is true, there will be no change in efficiency of the singlet oxygen reaction in D_2O compared with the efficiency in water.

Another effective technique for determining whether the reaction is Type I or Type II is to determine whether substrate and oxygen are competitive or not; in reactions in which the Type I reaction is much slower than Type II, there is no oxygen pressure dependence even at very low oxygen concentrations.[17, 18, 25] In a Type I reaction, there is often an oxygen presure dependence; oxygen may actually inhibit the reaction, although this is not the only possible behavior. These techniques have been used by McDonagh to establish that singlet oxygen is the intermediate in bilirubin photooxidation (page 56, this volume).

REFERENCES

1. Adams, D. R., and F. Wilkinson. Lifetime of singlet oxygen in liquid solution. J. Chem. Soc., Faraday Trans. 2, 68:586–593, 1972.
2. Ballou, D., G. Palmer, and V. Massey. Direct demonstration of superoxide anion production during the oxidation of reduced flavin and of its catalytic decomposition by erythrocuprein. Biochem. Biophys. Res. Commun. 36:898–904, 1969.
3. Bartholemew, R. F., and R. S. Davidson. Photosensitized oxidation of amines. J. Chem. Soc. D(18):1174–1175, 1970.
4. Bartlett, P. D., and A. P. Schaap. Stereospecific formation of 1,2-dioxetanes from *cis-* and *trans-*diethoxyethylenes by singlet oxygen. (Communication to the editor) J. Am. Chem. Soc. 92:3223–3225, 1970.
5. Bellin, J. S. Properties of pigments in the bound state: A review. Photochem. Photobiol. 4:33–44, 1965.
6. Berg, H., M. A. Gollmick, H. E. A. Kramer, and A. Maute. In Proceedings of the Sixth International Congress on Photobiology, Bochum, 1972. (In press)
7. Cohen, S. G., and A. D. Litt. Rate constants of interaction of benzophenone triplet with amines. Tetrahedron Lett. 11:837–840, 1970.
8. Foote, C. S. Mechanism of addition of singlet oxygen to olefins and other substrates. Pure Appl. Chem. 27:635–645, 1971.
9. Foote, C. S. Mechanisms of photosensitized oxidation. Science 162:963–970, 1968.
10. Foote, C. S. Photosensitized oxygenations and the role of singlet oxygen. Acc. Chem. Res. 1:104–110, 1968.
11. Foote, C. S., Y. C. Chang, and R. W. Denny. Chemistry of singlet oxygen. X. Carotenoid quenching parallels biological protection. (Communication to the editor) J. Am. Chem. Soc. 92:5216–5218, 1970.
12. Foote, C. S., and R. W. Denny. Chemistry of singlet oxygen. VII. Quenching by β-carotene. (Communication to the editor) J. Am. Chem. Soc. 90:6233–6235, 1968.
13. Foote, C. S., and J. W.-P. Lin. Chemistry of singlet oxygen. VI. Photooxygenation of enamines: Evidence for an intermediate. Tetrahedron Lett. 29:3267–3270, 1968.
14. Foote, C. S., and J. W. Peters. Photooxidation of sulfides, pp. 129–153. In Twenty-third International Congress of Pure and Applied Chemistry, Special Lectures, Vol. 4. London: Butterworths, 1971.
15. Foote, C. S., E. R. Peterson, and K-W. Lee. Chemistry of singlet oxygen. XVI. Long lifetime of singlet oxygen in carbon disulfide. (Communication to the editor) J. Am. Chem. Soc. 94:1032–1033, 1972.
16. Gmelin's Handbuch der anorganischen Chemie. (8th ed.) Verlag Chemie, 1958.
17. Gollnick, K. Type II photooxygenation reactions in solution. Adv. Photochem. 6:1–122, 1968.
18. Gollnick, K., and G. O. Schenck. Oxygen as a dienophile, pp. 255–344. In J. Hamer, Ed. 1,4-Cycloaddition Reactions. New York: Academic Press, Inc., 1967.
19. Higgins, R., C. S. Foote, and H. Cheng. Chemistry of singlet oxygen. V. Reactivity and kinetic characterization. Adv. Chem. Ser. No. 77:102–117, 1968.

20. Kasche, V., and L. Lindqvist. Transient species in the photochemistry of eosin. Photochem. Photobiol. 4:923–933, 1965.
21. Kearns, D. R. Physical and chemical properties of singlet molecular oxygen. Chem. Rev. 71:395–427, 1971.
22. Kepka, A. G., and L. I. Grossweiner. Photodynamic oxidation of iodide ion and aromatic amino acids by eosin. Photochem. Photobiol. 14:621–639, 1972.
23. Koizumi, M., and Y. Usui. Photooxidative bleaching of some dyes with oxygen via D–O and D–D mechanisms. In Proceedings of the Sixth International Congress on Photobiology, Bochum, 1972. (In press)
24. Krinsky, N. Function, pp. 669–716. In O. Isler, Ed. Carotenoids. Basel: Birkhäuser Verlag, 1971.
25. Livingston, R. Photochemical autoxidation, pp. 249–298. In W. O. Lundberg, Ed. Autoxidation and Antioxidants. Vol. I. New York: Interscience Publishers, 1961.
26. Mathews-Roth, M. M., and N. I. Krinsky. Studies on the protective functions of the carotenoid pigments of *Sarcina lutea*. Photochem. Photobiol. 11:419–428, 1970.
27. Mazur, S., and C. S. Foote. Chemistry of singlet oxygen. IX. A stable dioxetane from photooxygenation of tetramethoxyethylene. (Communication to the editor) J. Am. Chem. Soc. 92:3225–3226, 1970.
28. McCord, J. M., and I. Fridovich. The utility of superoxide dismutase in studying free radical reactions. II. The mechanism of the mediation of cytochrome *c* reduction by a variety of electron carriers. J. Biol. Chem. 245:1374–1377, 1970.
29. Merkel, P. B., and D. R. Kearns. Remarkable solvent effects on the lifetime of $^1\Delta_g$ oxygen. (Communication to the editor) J. Am. Chem. Soc. 94:1029–1030, 1972.
30. Merkel, P. B., R. Nilsson, and D. R. Kearns. Deuterium effects on singlet oxygen lifetimes in solutions. A new test of singlet oxygen reactions. (Communication to the editor) J. Am. Chem. Soc. 94:1030–1031, 1972.
31. Miller, R. W. Reactions of superoxide anion, catechols, and cytochrome *c*. Can. J. Biochem. 48:935–939, 1970.
32. Nemoto, M., Y. Usui, and M. Koizumi. The occurrence of a D–D mechanism in ethanolic solutions of eosine. Bull. Chem. Soc. Japan 40:1035–1040, 1967.
33. Nilsson, R., P. B. Merkel, and D. R. Kearns. Unambiguous evidence for the participation of singlet oxygen (1) in photodynamic oxidation of amino acids. Photochem. Photobiol. 16:117–124, 1972.
34. Saito, I., S. Kato, and T. Matsuura. Photoinduced reactions. XL. Addition of singlet oxygen to monocyclic ring. Tetrahedron Lett. 239–242, 1970.
35. Schenck, G. O., H.-D. Becker, K.-H. Schulte-Elte, and C. H. Krauch. Mit Benzophenon photosensibilisierte Autoxydation von sek. Alkoholen und Äthern. Darstellung von α-Hydroperoxyden. Chem. Ber. 96:509–516, 1963.
36. Schenck, G. O., and E. Koch. Zwischenreaktionen bei photosensibilisierten Prozessen in Losungen. Z. Elektrochem. 64:170–177, 1960.
37. Sherman, W. V., and S. G. Cohen. Flash photolysis of benzophenone in 2-propanol. Effect of phenyl disulfide. J. Phys. Chem. 70:178, 1966.
38. Smith, W. F., Jr. Kinetic evidence for both quenching and reaction of singlet oxygen with triethylamine in pyridine solution. J. Am. Chem. Soc. 94:186–190, 1972.
39. Spikes, J. D. Photodynamic action. Photophysiology 3:33–64, 1968.

40. Spikes, J. D. In Proceedings of the Sixth International Congress on Photobiology, Bochum, 1972. (In press)
41. Spikes, J. D., and R. Livingston. The molecular biology of photodynamic action: Sensitized photoautoxidations in biological systems. Adv. Radiat. Biol. 3:29–121, 1969.
42. Spikes, J. D., and M. L. MacKnight. Dye-sensitized photooxidation of proteins. Ann. N.Y. Acad. Sci. 171:149–161, 1970.
43. Spikes, J. D., and R. Straight. Sensitized photochemical processes in biological systems. Ann. Rev. Phys. Chem. 18:409–436, 1967.
44. Wilkinson, F. Progress in photobiology. In Proceedings of the Sixth International Congress on Photobiology, Bochum, 1972. (In press)
45. Youtsey, K. J., and L. I. Grossweiner. Optical excitation of the eosin-human serum albumin complex. Photochem. Photobiol. 6:721–731, 1967.

DAVID A. LIGHTNER

In Vitro Photooxidation Products of Bilirubin

In Vivo *Formation and Metabolism of Bilirubin*

The yellow, lipophilic bile pigment bilirubin IXα (Figure 1) is formed principally from the prosthetic heme group (Figure 1) of hemoglobin in the catabolism of red blood cells by a process that occurs normally in the reticuloendothelial cells of the liver, spleen, and bone marrow. Other hemoproteins may contribute approximately 20 percent of the bilirubin formed under physiologic conditions in man,[49] and a minor fraction of the hemoglobin is converted to metabolites other than bilirubin.[45, 46, 50] Although other portions—namely, iron and protein of the hemoglobin (hemoprotein) molecule—re-enter the metabolic pool, the heme is not reutilized but suffers rupture of its macrocyclic ring by specific oxidation on and in the region of the α-methene carbon. The oxidation is accomplished in several steps * by a mixed-function, micro-

---

This research was supported by the National Science Foundation (GP–32483X and GP–35699) and the National Institute of Child Health and Human Development, U.S. Public Health Service (HD–07358).

* These involve oxidation at the α-carbon to give an α-hydroxyheme Fe^{2+} followed by tautomerization to the α-oxophlorin Fe^{3+}. The latter adds oxygen (presumably ground-state oxygen), bridging the adjacent pyrrole rings and rearranging with expulsion of CO to give an Fe^{3+} biliverdin complex. Loss of iron leads to biliverdin.

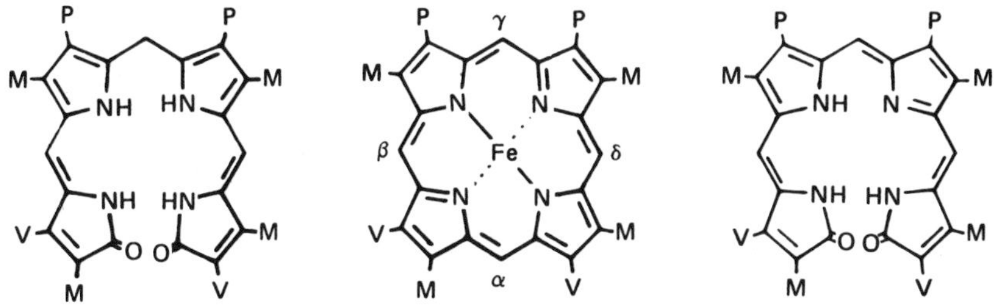

FIGURE 1 Structural formulas for bilirubin (1), hematin (2), and biliverdin (3).

somal heme oxygenase with resultant extrusion of CO (C of the α-methene bridge) and Fe^{3+} and subsequent formation of the green bile pigment biliverdin IXα (Figure 1).[49, 53] Biliverdin reductase converts biliverdin to bilirubin efficiently.

The excretion (hepatic transfer from blood to bile) of the toxic, lipophilic bilirubin is facilitated by its conversion principally to a water-soluble diglucuronide. Thus, the bilirubin that is carried in the plasma as an albumin complex (one albumin molecule effectively binds [17] and transports two bilirubin molecules) is transferred across the sinusoidal surface of the hepatocytes and into the cell after prior dissociation from albumin. The plasma membrane of the liver cells excludes the large, water-soluble albumin–bilirubin complex but is permeable to unbound lipophilic bilirubin. This transfer may be assisted by acceptor proteins in the hepatic cytoplasm,[1] but it clearly requires the bilirubin to become dissociated from albumin at the transfer site. Glucuronyl transferase and associated enzymes catalyze the esterification of the two propionic acid groups of bilirubin to their glucuronyl esters and thereby serve as the principal means of converting lipophilic, unconjugated bilirubin to a water-soluble conjugate, bilirubin diglucuronide. Other bilirubin conjugates—e.g., monoglucuronides, sulfates, acylglycosides of glucose and xylose, and disaccharides of hexuronic acids—have been reported but their functional importance is uncertain.[4] Bilirubin diglucuronide is secreted from the hepatic conjugating site into the bile, whence it enters the gut and is subject to further chemical change, usually hydrogenation, the nature of the change depending upon the presence and capabilities of the fecal flora.[10, 34] It is normally excreted in the feces in a highly reduced but optically active form, *l*-stercobilin(ogen).[10, 21, 33]

Hyperbilirubinemia of the Newborn—Causes and Treatment [2, 51]

The circulating, unconjugated, albumin-complexed bilirubin is present in normal human serum to the extent of 0.1–1.5 mg/100 ml.[47] However, the normal percentage of *unconjugated* bilirubin may be dramatically increased to dangerously high levels, 15–25 mg/100 ml or greater,[9, 14, 47] by at least three types of abnormalities: overproduction of bilirubin, inadequate hepatic uptake, and defective conjugation.[49, 50] *Conjugated* hyperbilirubinemia is usually caused by "regurgitation" of bilirubin diglucuronide into the plasma as a result of functional cholestasis, disruption of the hepatic architecture, or extrahepatic biliary obstruction.[50] However, it is *unconjugated* bilirubin that may cross the blood–brain barrier, gain access to the central nervous system, and lead to irreversible damage (kernicterus) with resultant retarded motor development, cerebral palsy, or even death. Other adverse metabolic effects associated with unconjugated hyperbilirubinemia include inhibition of DNA synthesis and stimulated CO_2 production from acetate in the liver and brain.[55]

Nearly all newborn infants show elevated levels of unconjugated bilirubin shortly after birth, but the concentration rarely exceeds 12 mg/100 ml in full-term infants and usually drops significantly during the first postnatal week.[54] However, even 12 mg/100 ml of unconjugated bilirubin may be a dangerously high level for the neonate, particularly when the albumin levels are low or the albumin-binding capacity is impaired. Moreover, if the major components of the bilirubin transport system—hepatic uptake, conjugation, and biliary excretion in the neonatal liver, which is functionally immature at birth—do not develop rapidly, the infant will suffer a continuing and increasing exposure to neurotoxic unconjugated bilirubin at levels exceeding the binding capacity of the existing albumin. Thus, neonatal hyperbilirubinemia can be an extremely dangerous condition.

Jaundice of the newborn has been treated successfully by complete blood transfusion to remove the excessive circulating bilirubin,[9, 45, 46, 49, 50] by administration of phenobarbital to stimulate hepatic uptake,[45, 46, 49–51, 57, 59] and by phototherapy to destroy the bilirubin and convert it into water-soluble, excretable products.[2, 27, 36, 40, 45, 46, 49–51] The phototherapy method was first reported by Cremer *et al.* in 1958 [7] and has since been increasingly applied.[2, 27, 36, 40, 49–51] However, there are many unanswered questions associated with this treatment, and it remains a controversial,[35] widely discussed procedure.[2, 5, 37, 39, 43–46, 49–51]

Phototherapy and Bilirubin

For whatever reasons the infant might be jaundiced at birth, available data [2, 37, 45, 46, 49] indicate that exposure of the neonate to sunlight or artificial blue or white light lowers the total serum bilirubin levels, especially unconjugated bilirubin; that the yellow coloration disappears from the irradiated *exposed* areas of the skin; and that a portion of the circulating bilirubin is excreted into the bile, urine, and feces as unknown but presumably water-soluble substances. One might therefore logically ask: What, specifically, does the light do, and are there any special light energies (wavelengths) that are more important than others for the success of the phototherapy? The answers to those questions have already been given in part. The light clearly stimulates a lowering of serum bilirubin levels, and it also appears to convert the bilirubin into water-soluble derivatives (but apparently not bilirubin glucuronides). The most effective wavelengths of light in this process are in the visible region of the spectrum, roughly between 400 and 500 nm.[52] Light emission farther into the red is either much less effective or ineffective, but emission in the ultraviolet may be effective. However, in regard to the latter, the process of exposing the infant to ultraviolet irradiation has potential side effects inherent in it and should be approached with extreme apprehension.[56]

How does the light act to lower serum bilirubin levels? The primary process in the phototherapy doubtless involves light absorption by bilirubin. It is not surprising therefore that 400–500-nanometer light is most effective and coincides with the 440–460-nanometer absorption band of bilirubin (Figure 2). The breadth of this band, whose wings extend to 400 and 500 nm, suggests that any light emitted from an external source in that region will be absorbed to some extent. Light at longer wavelengths, i.e., beyond the 440–460-nanometer absorption band of bilirubin, will not be absorbed and should therefore be ineffective. However, light at shorter wavelengths may be absorbed by the higher energy absorption bands ($\lambda \sim 300$ and 230 nm) of bilirubin. The efficiency and product distribution of *in vitro* photolysis of bilirubin at the absorption bands mentioned is under investigation in our laboratories. However, the matters of special interest in connection with jaundice phototherapy are the biochemistry associated with light absorption in the vicinity of the long-wavelength electronic transition (440–460 nm) and the consequent promotion of bilirubin to its lowest excited state.

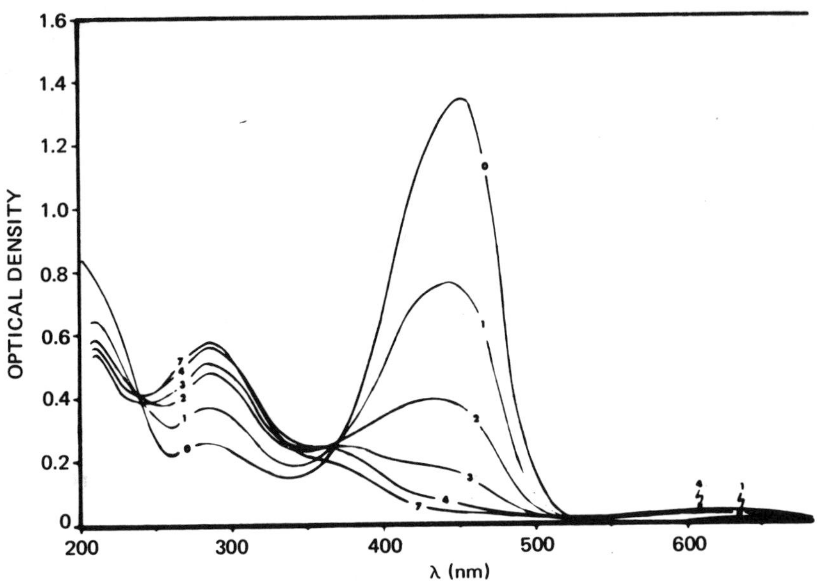

FIGURE 2 Visible-ultraviolet spectral curves of bilirubin (0.4 m*M* in methanol plus a trace of NH_4OH) at time 0 h and at various reaction times (h) during its photooxygenation. All spectra are run after a concentration dilution of 1 : 22.5. The photooxygenation was carried out in a Pyrex water-cooled immersion apparatus with which a Sylvania 500 Q/CL, 500-W tungsten–halogen lamp was used. (From Lightner *et al.*[20] Reprinted by permission.)

The Fate of Bilirubin

What is the fate of bilirubin in its lowest excited state?

1. McDonagh has shown that excited-state bilirubin is a singlet oxygen ($^1O_2$) sensitizer.[6, 31] However, it is apparently not as efficient a sensitizer as, for example, methylene blue and hematoporphyrin. Nonetheless, the lowest-singlet excited-state bilirubin (~ 63 kcal/mol) would appear to undergo intersystem crossing to a triplet excited state that transfers energy and inverts electron spin in triplet ground-state oxygen to product–singlet oxygen, presumably $^1\Delta_g$.[12] Singlet oxygen is thought to be responsible for tissue damage in porphyria.[29]

2. Excited-state bilirubin has also been shown (*in vitro*) to add hydroxylic solvents to its vinyl groups.[28] Thus, bilirubin could conceivably add water, sulfhydryl, hydroxyl, or perhaps even amino groups of cellular proteins. However, such photochemical additions to the reactive vinyl groups do not destroy the bilirubin chromophore and as such may not be

directly responsible for the disappearance of bilirubin from the skin of exposed infants. Nonetheless, if the bilirubin were rendered water-soluble by this type of conjugation with the vinyl groups, its excretion might be facilitated.

3. Excited-state bilirubin might isomerize to a more rapidly excreted form.

4. Excited-state bilirubin could transfer all or some its energy to other substrates, thereby inducing a special reactivity leading to its elimination. In photosynthesis of blue-green and red algae, energy transfer from biliproteins to chlorophyll is known to occur.[32] However, energy transfer from bilirubin has not been extensively reported.

With the belief that an important mechanism for the lowering of serum bilirubin levels is closely tied to the photooxygenation of bilirubin, I now address myself to that phenomenon.

Photooxygenation In Vitro

Following the observations of Ostrow *et al.*[42] that aqueous alkaline solutions of bilirubin were unstable during illumination, we initiated our bilirubin photooxidation studies in water or methanol solvents, using sufficient ammonia to dissolve the bilirubin. However, when we became interested in jaundice phototherapy, it was necessary to determine whether oxygen was required for the *in vitro* photodestruction of bilirubin. A carefully deoxygenated aqueous ammonia solution of bilirubin was thus photolyzed for a period of 72 h under nitrogen.* In the workup a substantial amount (30%) of bilirubin was recovered by preparative thin-layer chromatography (TLC), and the remaining products were mainly green, blue-green, pink, and violet pigments. In contrast, *oxygenated* aqueous or methanolic ammonia solutions of bilirubin were rapidly photodegraded, as shown in Figure 2.† The photooxygenation reaction was markedly accelerated by the addition of known singlet-oxygen ($^1O_2$) sensitizers, e.g., methylene blue or rose bengal. McDonagh then demonstrated that $^1O_2$ was indeed involved in the photodegradation and showed that bilirubin is a $^1O_2$ sensitizer, albeit an inefficient one.[31] These findings were recently confirmed by Bonnett and Stewart.[6] It would appear, therefore, that bilirubin may sensitize its own photode-

* Hanovia 8A36, 100-W, medium-pressure mercury lamp. Water-cooled Pyrex immersion well apparatus.

† Concentrations varied but were usually ~ 1.5 mM in bilirubin and 18 mM in NH_3. Some NH_3 is doubtless removed for solutions by the oxygen flow. In a control reaction without light, 91 percent of bilirubin was isolated from a methanolic ammonia solution oxygenated for 20 h.

struction *in vitro,* and we assume that such a phenomenon might also occur *in vivo* for bilirubin deposited in the cutaneous tissues of the jaundiced neonate. Presumably, the oxygen necessary for the *in vivo* photodegradation diffuses into the skin from the air or is supplied by the circulatory system. We do not know of any studies relating atmospheric oxygen concentration and the efficacy of the phototherapy method.

Reaction of Bilirubin with $^1O_2$*: The Potential Intermediates*

Several well-known types of reactions of $^1O_2$ with organic substrates are depicted in Figure 3. They include the "ene" reaction, a Diels–Alder reaction involving 1,4-addition of $^1O_2$ leading to an *endo*-peroxide (intermediate), and reaction of electron-rich carbon–carbon double bonds leading to products via a dioxetane intermediate from 1,2-addition of $^1O_2$.[12] Accordingly, one might logically examine the structure of bilirubin for the various sites where these "type" reactions might occur. Drawing from literature examples, McDonagh [31] first suggested that bilirubin might photodegrade by attack of $^1O_2$ at two sites: the vinyl groups and the enamine-like bridges (a and c) [structures (4) and (5) of Figure 4].

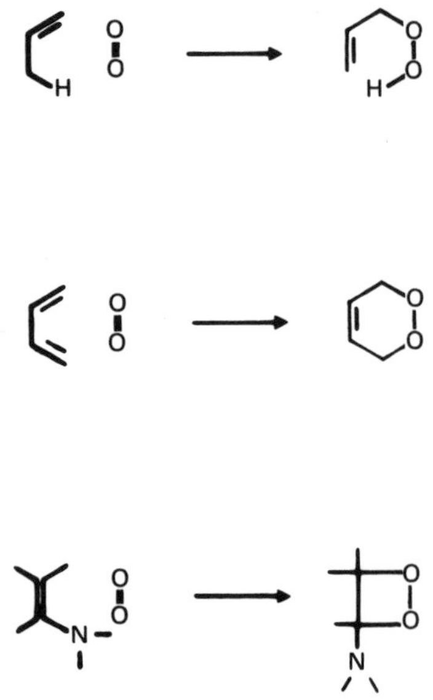

FIGURE 3 Three characteristic reactions of singlet oxygen. *Top:* "Ene" reaction. *Center:* Diels–Alder reaction. *Bottom:* Addition to electron-rich double bond (enamine).

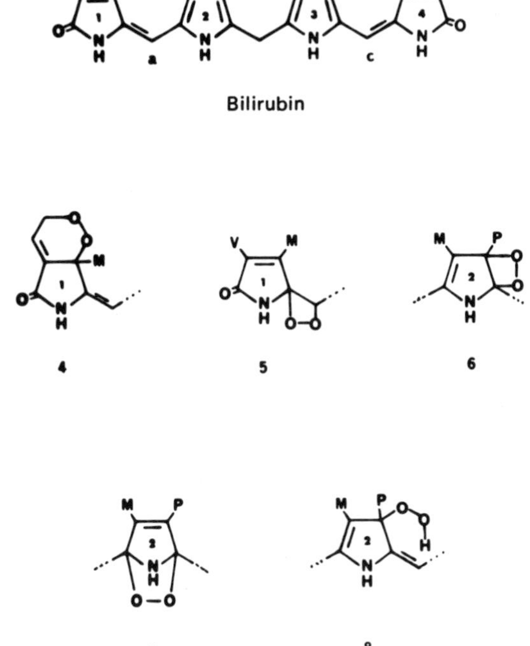

FIGURE 4 Structural formulas for some of the possible reaction intermediates of bilirubin with singlet oxygen following reactions of the type shown in Figure 3.

In an extension of this reasoning and by making further use of the $^1O_2$ reactions shown in Figure 3, a dioxetane intermediate might be conceptualized for the carbon–carbon double bonds of the central pyrrole rings (2 and 3) as depicted in structure (6). Furthermore, 1,4-addition of $^1O_2$ to those same pyrrole rings generates *endo*-peroxide structures such as structure (7). The possible products of the "ene" reaction (Figure 3) are many, and we suggest just one, structure (8), as shown. The implications of such sites of attack by $^1O_2$ on bilirubin and the fate of the structures indicated are examined in the following section.

Reaction of Bilirubin with $^1O_2$*: The Products*

1,4-Addition of $^1O_2$ to the vinyl groups of protoporphyrin IX with subsequent rearrangement to isolatable hydroxy-aldehydes is shown in Fig-

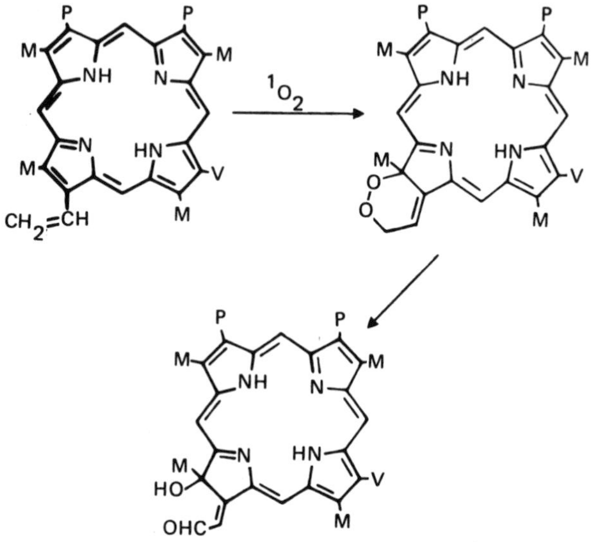

FIGURE 5 Diagram of reaction of singlet oxygen with a vinyl group of protoporphyrin IX.

ure 5.[16] Should such a reaction occur with bilirubin, the expected products would be the corresponding hydroxy-aldehydes (Figure 6). We have not as yet detected any hydroxy-aldehyde products of the general type indicated; however, the stability of such types of compounds is unknown, and they cannot be ruled out as "early" photoproducts. The reaction of $^1O_2$ at an enamine double bond is well known from the work of Foote and Lin,[13] who have shown that carbonyl products result from collapse of a dioxetane intermediate (Figure 7). When McDonagh applied this precedent to bilirubin,[31] he postulated as products methylvinyl-

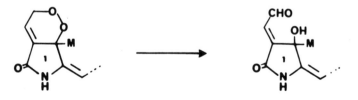

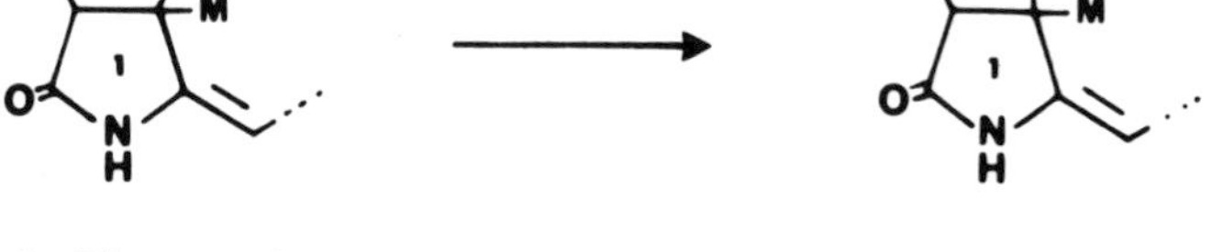

FIGURE 6 Diagram of proposed reaction of singlet oxygen with a vinyl group of bilirubin.

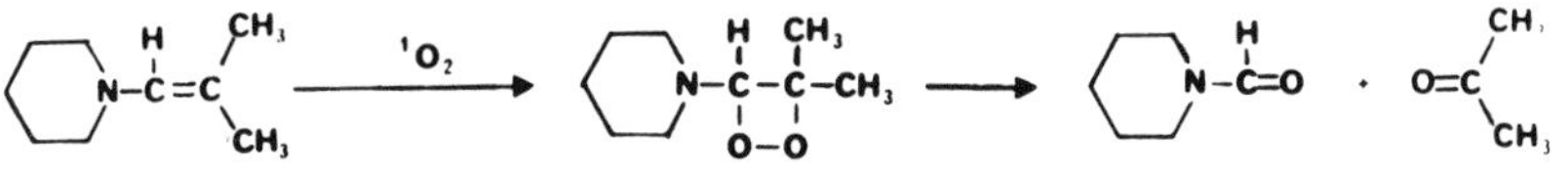

FIGURE 7 Diagram of reaction of singlet oxygen with an enamine double bond.

maleimide and a tripyrrolic aldehyde [structures (9) and (10) of Figure 8] or, as a consequence of a second reaction of this type, a dipyrrolic dialdehyde [structure (11)] composed of the two original, central rings of bilirubin. Thus, although several potential products are revealed from two of the analogies presented in the foregoing, to date we have not isolated any hydroxy-aldehyde photoproducts of the type suggested, nor have we isolated any di- or tripyrrolic aldehydes that might arise from the "enamine" reaction.

Even before these possibilities were suggested,[31] we were at work isolating and determining structures of the bilirubin photooxidation products with special emphasis on methylvinylmaleimide and hematinic acid. We reasoned that these might represent stable photoproducts, but we slowly became aware of the special lability of methylvinylmaleimide. Thus, our very early attempts to find methylvinylmaleimide were not at all successful, and we were concerned that the vinyl groups were particularly reactive [structure (4) of Figure 4] toward oxidation. To test this notion, we constructed a model compound that is structurally similar

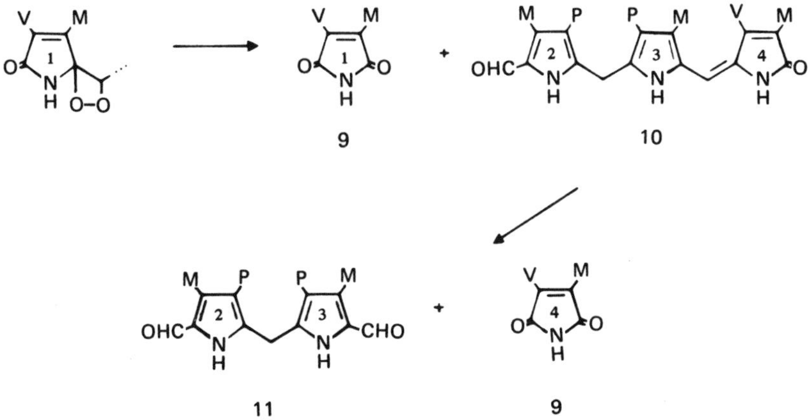

FIGURE 8 Structural formulas of proposed reaction products of singlet oxygen at the enamine-like double bonds of bilirubin via dioxetane intermediates.

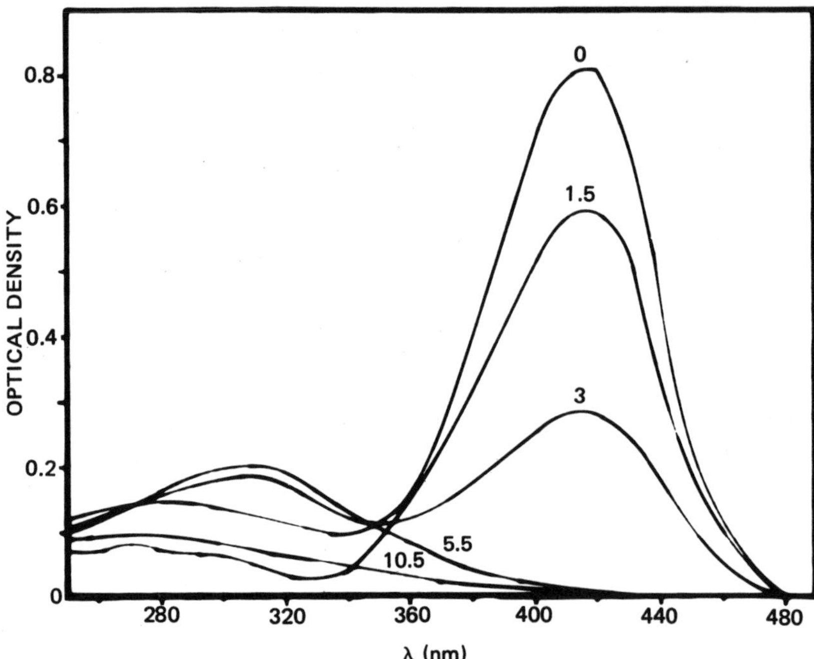

FIGURE 9 Visible-ultraviolet spectral curves of 5′-oxo-3′,4,4′-triethyl-3,5-dimethyl-1′,5′-dihydro-(2,2′)-dipyrrylmethene (0.55 m*M* in methanol) at time 0 h and at various reaction times (h) during its photooxygenation. All spectra are run after a concentration–dilution of 1 : 16, then 2 : 3. The photooxygenation was carried out in a Pyrex water-cooled immersion apparatus with which a Sylvania 500 Q/CL, 500-W tungsten–halogen lamp was used.

to one half of bilirubin and has a comparable visible-ultraviolet spectrum (Figure 9). In fact, it is structurally and spectroscopically reminiscent of Fischer's bilirubinic acids.[11] This dipyrrolic model compound [structure (12) of Figure 10] has no vinyl groups, and the two rings are distinguishable (as possible imide precursors) by virtue of their different sets of β-substituents. In the absence of added known $^1O_2$ sensitizers, methanolic solutions of the model compound underwent the spectral alterations shown in Figure 9. The rate of change was accelerated with added rose bengal. We surmise that the model compound is a weak $^1O_2$ sensitizer, as is bilirubin.

The products of photooxidation of the model compound were isolated by preparative TLC and the structures proved by spectroscopic methods.[23] The major products isolated were xeronimide and methoxylactam [struc-

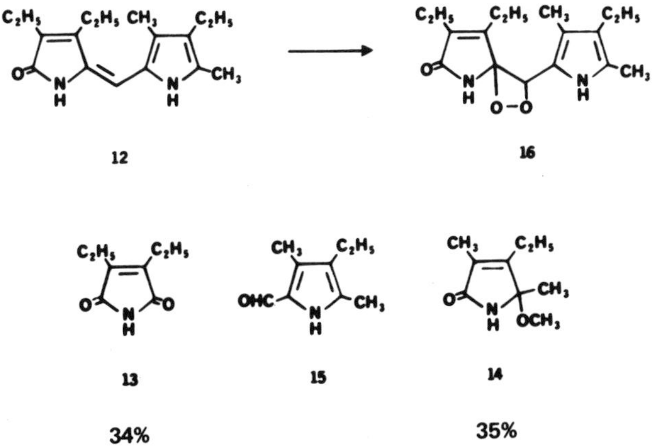

FIGURE 10 Diagram of a photooxygenation reaction of 5′-oxo-3′,4,4′-triethyl-3,5-dimethyl-1,5′-dihydro-(2,2′)-dipyrrylmethene (12) involving a dioxetane intermediate (16) and leading to monopyrrole products (13) and (14) in methanol.

tures (13) and (14), respectively, of Figure 10]. We could not find the expected kryptopyrrole aldehyde, structure (15), which was the aldehyde product anticipated from normal cleavage (see Figure 7) of dioxetane [structure (16)]. We therefore examined the rose bengal-sensitized photooxidation of structure (15) and discovered that it was smoothly and efficiently converted into structure (14).[26] We conclude therefore that methoxylactum arises as a secondary photoproduct and suggest that tri- or dipyrrolic aldehydes [structures (10) and (11)], should they be formed, might not be found as such following bilirubin photooxidation but would undergo rapid photooxidation to new products.

The photooxidative enamine cleavage was also demonstrated with mesobilirubin [structure (17)], from which we isolated methylethylmaleimide (Figure 11).[23] Here again, the problem of the vinyl group reactivity was circumvented as mesobilirubin has ethyl, rather than vinyl, groups. However, the generality of this type of reaction was confirmed when methylvinylmaleimide was isolated after careful and rapid workup from both bilirubin[23, 24] and biliverdin[18] either with or without added rose bengal.

The possibility of a third type of $^1O_2$ reaction of bilirubin—one proceeding via 1,4-addition to the central pyrrole rings [structure (7) of Figure 4]—was examined. Looking for a precedent, we searched for sensitized photooxidations of monopyrroles and discovered that very little information had been reported. The first report of a product-isola-

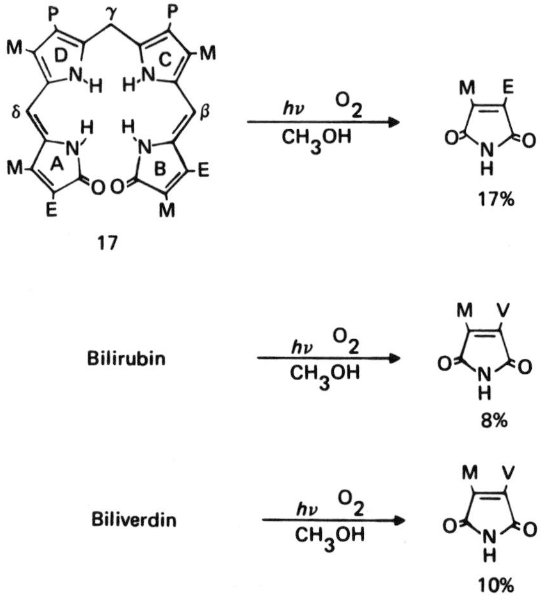

FIGURE 11 Diagram showing imide photooxidation products from mesobilirubin, bilirubin, and biliverdin.

tion of pyrrole itself appeared in 1939,[3] but it was not until the work of DeMayo and Reid [8] that the structure of that photoproduct was proved (Figure 12). The same authors suggested an *endo*-peroxide precursor to their isolated hydroxy-lactam. We found that we could repeat the reaction and that one mole equivalent of oxygen is quite rapidly consumed during the photooxygenation. The products from photooxidation in methanol are shown in Figure 13.[48] It may be noted that these products doubtless arise from pyrrole *endo*-peroxide, which may react with solvent or undergo internal structural reorganization.

Seeking a better model for the central two rings of bilirubin, we examined the rose bengal-sensitized photooxidation of 3,4-diethyl-2,5-dimethylpyrrole [structure (18)] in methanol and isolated and proved the structures of the major photoproducts.[25] (See Figure 14.) It was surprising to discover that either of the methyl groups or both may be lost to give methoxylactam and imide [structures (20) and (19), respectively]. Those products appear to arise from the anticipated *endo*-peroxide intermediate [structure (21)]. In addition, we have evidence for a dioxetane intermediate [structure 22)] in the isolated products [structures (23) and (24)], which can only arise by cleavage of the

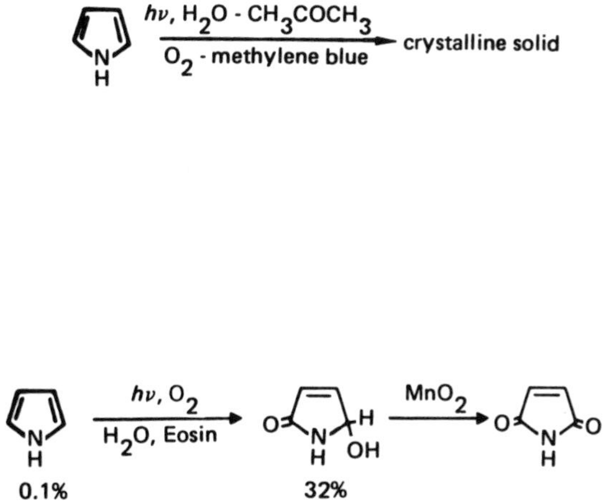

FIGURE 12 Diagram of two reported dye-sensitized photooxidations of pyrrole in aqueous solvent.

enamine-like double bonds of pyrrole. Whether the dioxetane intermediate is formed by 1,2-addition of $^1O_2$ or by rearrangement of *endo*-peroxide (21) is not established. Evidence for even further oxidation is found in structure (25).

The formation of imide and methoxylactam suggests that bilirubin *endo*-peroxide [structure (7) of Figure 15] might undergo analogous

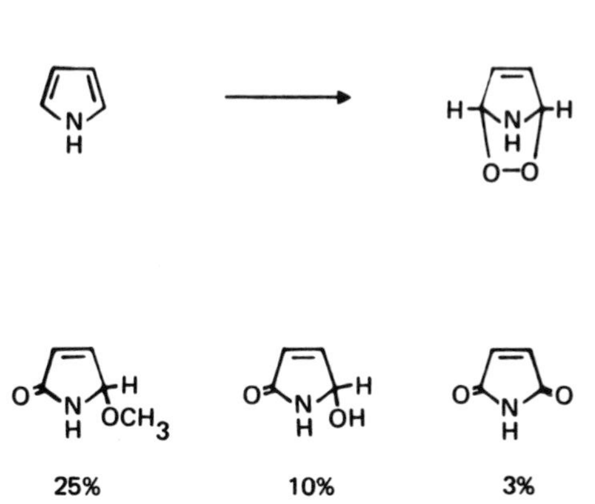

FIGURE 13 Diagram of the rose bengal-sensitized photooxygenation of pyrrole (methanol solvent) involving an *endo*-peroxide intermediate and leading to lactam and imide products.

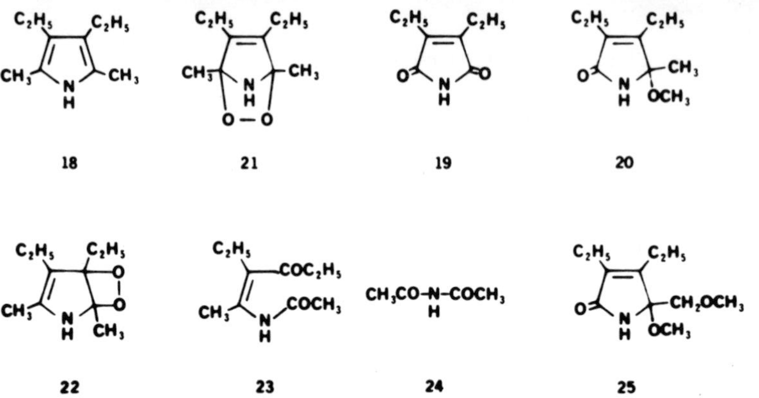

FIGURE 14 Structural formulas for the products (19), (20), (23), (24), and (25) and proposed intermediates (21) and (22) from rose bengal-sensitized photooxygenation of 3,4-diethyl-2,5-dimethylpyrrole in methanol.

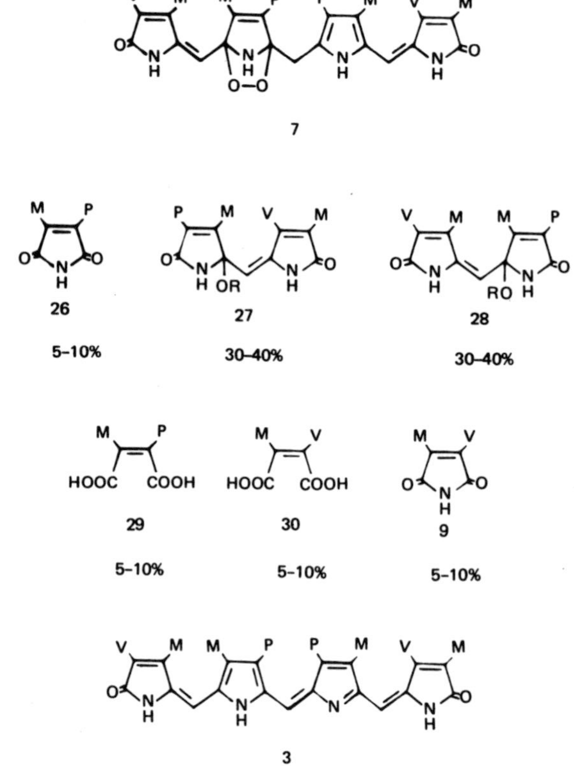

FIGURE 15 Structural formulas for the photooxygenation products of bilirubin and an *endo*-peroxide intermediate.

reactions leading to hematinic acid [structure (26)] and methoxy or hydroxy propentdyopents (depending on solvent) [structures (27) and (28)]. In fact, all of these, structures (26)–(28), were found,[22] in addition to methylvinylmaleimide (9), when either an aqueous or methanolic ammonia solution of bilirubin was photooxidized with or without added rose bengal-sensitizer.* In addition, in aqueous solvent, imide hydrolysis products [structures (29) and (30)] were obtained. Some biliverdin is also isolated. In keeping with these findings, if one re-examines the visible-ultraviolet spectral decomposition curves taken during bilirubin photooxidation (Figure 2), the appearance of weak biliverdin absorption maxima near 650 and 370 nm may be noted. Furthermore, the emergence of a relatively strong absorption maximum near 290 nm may be assigned to the propentdyopents (27) and (28). The major new absorptions that appear during bilirubin photooxygenation are therefore taken into account in addition to the structures of the major photoproducts produced in hydroxylic solvents.

The Formation of Biliverdin and Its Photooxidation

Biliverdin was one of the earliest suspected photoproducts of bilirubin,[38, 42] as suggested by the observation that bilirubin solutions exhibited a transient green coloration during photooxidation.[15, 58] Questions as to whether biliverdin is the primary photoproduct of bilirubin photooxidation and whether it is also the precursor to all other bilirubin products have arisen.[15, 23, 41, 58] We have shown that biliverdin is a product of bilirubin photooxidation, and that it is *not* the precursor to the majority of the isolated monopyrrole and dipyrrole photoproducts (Figure 15) formed in protic solvents.[20] If one examines the rate of biliverdin formation and compares it with the rate of bilirubin destruction during photooxidation in methanol, it may be concluded (Figure 16) that bilirubin photodegrades at a much faster rate than does biliverdin. Furthermore, the rate of bilirubin photodestruction is slowed somewhat by the increased concentration of biliverdin. This observation is in keeping with McDonagh's finding that biliverdin is a $^1O_2$ quencher.[30] At the proper reaction time, as much as a 16-percent yield of biliverdin may be isolated from photooxidation of bilirubin in methanol; in chloroform solvent, we have isolated biliverdin in a 38-percent yield.[20]

Just how the biliverdin is formed is not yet understood. It might arise initially from the "ene" reaction [structure (1) of Figure 3] near the

* Westinghouse or Sylvania tungsten–halogen lamp, 500-W, 500 Q/CL. Water-cooled Pyrex immersion well apparatus.

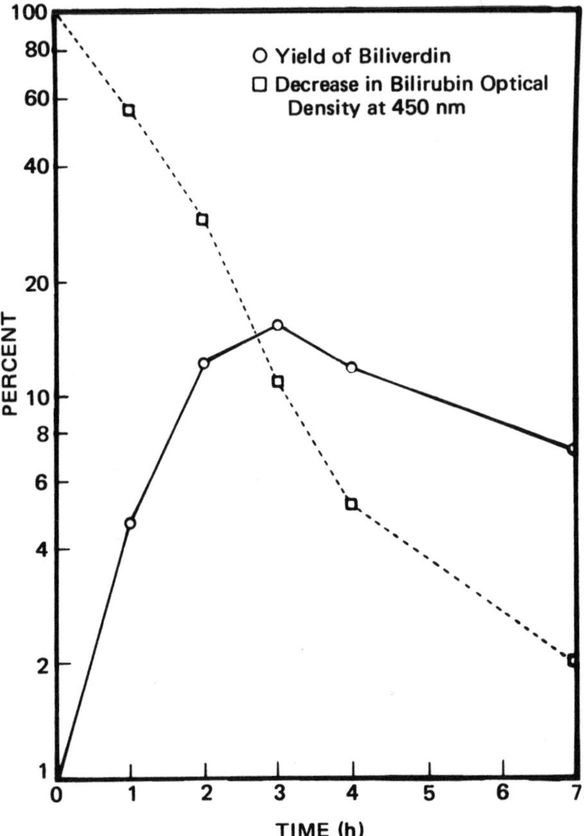

FIGURE 16 Yield (percentage) of biliverdin at various times of photooxygenation of bilirubin and decrease in optical density (100% at 0 h) of bilirubin versus time of photooxygenation. (From Lightner *et al.*[20] Reprinted by permission.)

central methylene bridge of bilirubin [structure (8) of Figure 4] to give first a hydroperoxide (Figure 17) that undergoes deprotonation at nitrogen and elimination of hydroperoxide ion. Alternatively, a radical reaction initiated by triplet sensitizer could lead to hydrogen abstraction at the central methylene bridge followed by reaction of that radical with oxygen. More work needs to be done on the reaction mechanism.

Finally, it is of some interest to note that photooxidation of biliverdin

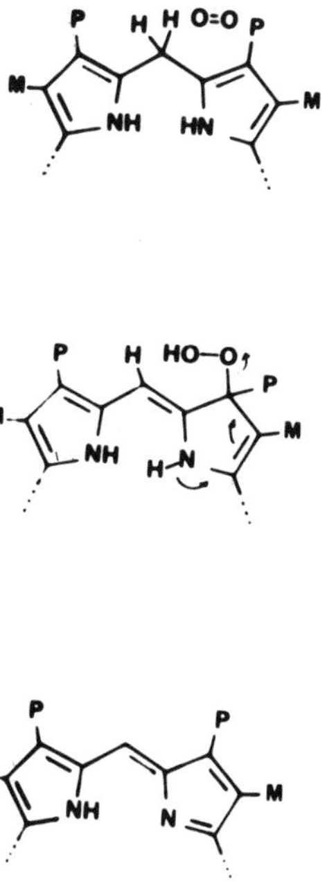

FIGURE 17 Structural formulas in a possible reaction sequence for the formation of biliverdin from bilirubin involving singlet oxygen.

is pH-sensitive. We have found the rate of photodestruction of biliverdin (as measured by decrease of the 375-nm absorption) to be 2–3 times faster at pH 7–8 than at pH 5. In addition, the rate of photooxidation of biliverdin in methanol is virtually the same as that of biliverdin dimethyl ester. Our preliminary results on the isolation and structure proof of the biliverdin photooxidation products (methanol solvent) include methylvinylmaleimide (9) [18] as previously noted, hematinic acid [structure (26)], and one of the isomeric methoxypropentdyopents [structure (28)].[19] (See Figure 18.)

Acknowledgments

The author appreciates the conscientious research efforts of Dr. Gary B. Quistad and Mr. Dave C. Crandall, who contributed so vitally to the success of this work. He is grateful to Ms. Theodora Nikos for assistance in compiling this work and to Ms. Elizabeth Irwin for assistance in obtaining high-resolution mass spectra.

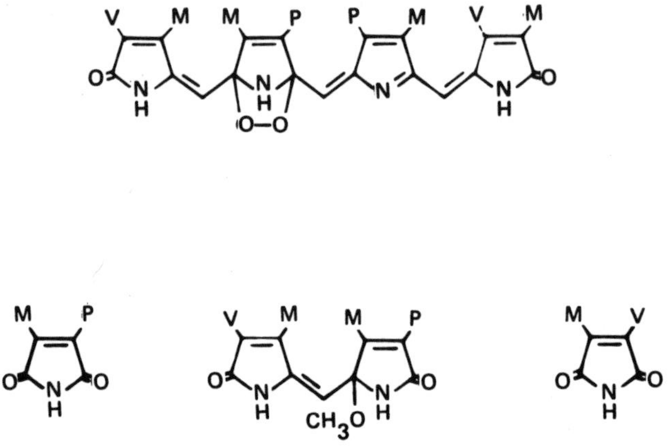

FIGURE 18 Some products from the photooxygenation of biliverdin and an *endo*-peroxide intermediate.

REFERENCES

1. Arias, I. M. Transfer of bilirubin from blood bile. Semin. Hematol. 9:55–70, 1972.
2. Bergsma, D., D. Y.-Y. Hsia, and C. Jackson, Eds. Bilirubin metabolism in the newborn. Birth Defects 6:1–136, 1970.
3. Bernheim, F., and J. E. Morgan. Photo-oxidation of pyrrhole. Nature 144:290, 1939.
4. Billing, B. H., and F. H. Jansen. Enigma of bilirubin conjugation. Gastroenterology 61:258–260, 1971.
5. Blue light and jaundice. Br. Med. J. 2:5–6, 1970.
6. Bonnett, R., and J. C. M. Stewart. Singlet oxygen in the photooxidation of bilirubin in hydroxylic solvents. Biochem. J. 130: 895–897, 1972.
7. Cremer, R. J., P. W. Perryman, and D. H. Richards. Influence of light on the hyperbilirubinaemia of infants. Lancet 1:1094–1097, 1958.
8. DeMayo, P., and S. T. Reid. The photo-oxidation of pyrrole: A simple synthesis of maleimide. Chem. Ind. (Lond.) [no vol.] 1576–1577, 1962.
9. Diamond, L. K. A history of jaundice in the newborn. Birth Defects 6:3–6, 1970.
10. Elder, G., C. H. Gray, and D. C. Nicholson. Bile pigment fate in gastrointestinal tract. Semin. Hematol. 9:71–89, 1972.
11. Fischer, H., and H. Orth. Die Chemie des Pyrrols, p. 126, Vol. 2. Leipzig: Akademische Velagsgesellschaft, 1934.
12. Foote, C. S. Mechanisms of photosensitized oxidation. Science 162:963–970, 1968.
13. Foote, C. S., and J. W.-P. Lin. Chemistry of singlet oxygen. VI. Photooxygenation of enamines: Evidence for an intermediate. Tetrahedron Lett. 29:3267–3270, 1968.

14. Gellis, S. S. The use of increased light as routine prophylaxis for hyperbilirubinemia of the low-birthweight infant. Birth Defects 6:90–92, 1970.
15. Gray, C. H., A. Kulczycka, and D. C. Nicholson. The photodecomposition of bilirubin and other bile pigments. J. Chem. Soc. [Perkin I] 3:288–294, 1972.
16. Inhoffen, H. H., H. Brockmann, Jr., and K.-M. Bliesener. Photoprotoporphyrinie und ihre Umwandlung in Spirographis-sowie Isospirographis-porphyrin. Justus Liebigs Ann. Chem. 730:173, 1969.
17. Jacobsen, J. Binding of bilirubin to human serum albumin—or determination of the dissociation constants. FEBS Lett. 5:112–114, 1969.
18. Lightner, D. A., and D. C. Crandall. Biliverdin photo-oxidation. *In vitro* formation of methylvinylmaleimide. FEBS Lett. 20:53–56, 1972.
19. Lightner, D. A., and D. C. Crandall. The photooxygenation of biliverdin [bilirubin; jaundice phototherapy; singlet oxygen; hematinic acid; propentdyopents]. Tetrahedron Lett. 953–956, 1973.
20. Lightner, D. A., D. C. Crandall, S. Gertler, and G. B. Quistad. On the formation of biliverdin during photooxygenation of bilirubin *in vitro.* FEBS Lett. 30:309–312, 1973.
21. Lightner, D. A., E. L. Docks, J. Horwitz, and A. Moscowitz. Circular dichroism studies at variable temperature: Urobilinoid conformation. Proc. Natl. Acad. Sci. (USA) 67:1361–1366, 1970.
22. Lightner, D. A., and G. B. Quistad. Hematinic acid and propentdyopents from bilirubin photo-oxidation *in vitro.* FEBS Lett. 25: 94–96, 1972.
23. Lightner, D. A., and G. B. Quistad. Imide products from photooxidation of bilirubin and mesobilirubin. Nature New Biol. 236:203–205, 1972.
24. Lightner, D. A., and G. B. Quistad. Methylvinylmaleimide from bilirubin photooxidation. Science 175:324, 1972.
25. Lightner, D. A., and G. B. Quistad. Photooxidation of 3,4-diethyl-2,5-dimethylpyrrole. Angew. Chem. (Int. ed.) 11:215–216, 1972.
26. Lightner, D. A., and G. B. Quistad. The dye-sensitized photooxygenation of pyrrole α-aldehyde. J. Heterocyclic Chem. 10: 273–274, 1973.
27. Lucey, J. F. Neonatal phototherapy: Uses, problems, and questions. Semin. Hematol. 9:127–135, 1972.
28. Manitto, P., and D. Monti. Photoaddition of sulphydryl groups to bilirubin *in vitro*. Experientia 28:379–380, 1972.
29. Mathews-Roth, M. M., M. A. Pathak, T. B. Fitzpatrick, L. C. Harber, and E. H. Kass. Beta-carotene as a photoprotective agent in erythropoietic protoporphyria. N. Engl. J. Med. 282:1231–1234, 1970.
30. McDonagh, A. F. Evidence for singlet oxygen quenching by biliverdin IX-α dimethyl ester and its relevance to bilirubin photo-oxidation. Biochem. Biophys. Res. Commun. 48:408–415, 1972.
31. McDonagh, A. F. The role of singlet oxygen in bilirubin photo-oxidation. Biochem. Biophys. Res. Commun. 44:1306–1311, 1971.
32. Miedziejko, E., and D. Frackowiak. Excitation energy transfer in bilirubin–chlorophyll aggregates. Photochem. Photobiol. 10:97–108, 1969.
33. Moscowitz, A., W. C. Krueger, I. T. Kay, G. Skewes, and S. Bruckenstein. On the origin of the optical activity in the urobilins. Proc. Natl. Acad. Sci. (USA) 52:1190–1194, 1964.
34. Moscowitz, A., M. Weimer, D. A. Lightner, Z. J. Petryka, E. Davis, and C. J. Watson. The *in vitro* conversion of bile pigments to the urobilinoids

by a rat Clostridia species as compared with the human fecal flora. III. Natural *d*-urobilin, synthetic *i*-urobilin, and synthetic *i*-urobilinogen. Biochem. Med. 4:149–164, 1970.

35. Odell, G. B., R. S. Brown, and N. A. Holtzman. Dye-sensitized photooxidation of albumin associated with a decreased capacity for protein-binding of bilirubin. Birth Defects 6:31–35, 1970.
36. Ostrow, J. D. Mechanisms of bilirubin photodegradation. Semin. Hematol. 9:113–125, 1972.
37. Ostrow, J. D. Photochemical and biochemical basis of the treatment of neonatal jaundice. Prog. Liver Dis. 4:447–462, 1972.
38. Ostrow, J. D. Photo-oxidative derivatives of [^{14}C] bilirubin and their excretion by the Gunn rat, pp. 117–127. In I. A. D. Bouchier and B. H. Billing, Eds. Bilirubin Metabolism. Oxford: Blackwell Scientific Publications, 1967.
39. Ostrow, J. D. Recent advances in bilirubin metabolism. Viewpoints Dig. Dis. 3:1–4, 1971.
40. Ostrow, J. D., and R. V. Branham. Photodecay of bilirubin *in vitro* and in the jaundiced (Gunn) rat. Birth Defects 6:93–99, 1970.
41. Ostrow, J. D., and R. V. Branham. Photodecomposition of bilirubin and biliverdin *in vitro*. Gastroenterology 58:15–25, 1970.
42. Ostrow, J. D., L. Hammaker, and R. Schmid. The preparation of crystalline bilirubin-C^{14}. J. Clin. Invest. 40:1442–1452, 1961.
43. Phototherapy and hyperbilirubinemia. J. Pediatr. 74:989–990, 1969.
44. Phototherapy for neonatal jaundice. Lancet 1:825–826, 1970.
45. Physiology and disorders of hemoglobin degradation. Semin. Hematol. I. 9:1–106, 1972.
46. Physiology and disorders of hemoglobin degradation. Semin. Hematol. II. 9:107–224, 1972.
47. Powell, L. W. Clinical aspects of unconjugated hyperbilirubinemia. Semin. Hematol. 9:91–105, 1972.
48. Quistad, G. B., and D. A. Lightner. Pyrrole photooxidation. Direct formation of maleimides. J. Chem. Soc. D. 18:1099–1100, 1971.
49. Schmid, R. Bilirubin metabolism in man. N. Engl. J. Med. 287:703–709, 1972.
50. Schmid, R. Hyperbilirubinemia, pp. 871–902. In J. B. Stanbury, J. B. Wyngaarden, and D. S. Fredrickson, Eds. The Metabolic Basis of Inherited Disease (2nd ed.). New York: McGraw-Hill Book Co., Inc., 1966.
51. Schmid, R. More light on neonatal hyperbilirubinemia? N. Engl. J. Med. 285:520–522, 1971.
52. Sisson, T. R. C., D. Kendall, R. E. Davies, and D. Berger. Factors influencing the effectiveness of phototherapy in neonatal hyperbilirubinemia. Birth Defects 6:100–105, 1970.
53. Tenhunen, R. The enzymatic degradation of heme. Semin. Hematol. 9:19–29, 1972.
54. Thaler, M. M. Neonatal hyperbilirubinemia. Semin. Hematol. 9:107–112, 1972.
55. Thaler, M. M. Toxic effects of bilirubin and its photodecomposition products. Birth Defects 6:128–130, 1970.
56. Urbach, F., Ed. International Conference on the Biologic Effects of Ultraviolet Radiation (with Emphasis on the Skin), 1st, Rutgers University, 1966. Proceedings. Oxford: Pergamon Press, 1969.

57. Valaes, T., S. Petmezaki, and S. A. Doxiadis. Effect on neonatal hyperbilirubinemia of phenobarbital during pregnancy or after birth: Practical value of the treatment in a population with high risk of unexplained severe neonatal jaundice. Birth Defects 6:46–54, 1970.
58. Velapoldi, R. A., and O. Menis. Formation and stabilities of free bilirubin and bilirubin complexes with transition and rare-earth elements. Clin. Chem. 17:1165–1170, 1971.
59. Yaffe, S. J., C. S. Catz, L. Stern, and G. Levy. The use of phenobarbital in neonatal jaundice. Birth Defects 6:37–44, 1970.

ANTONY F. McDONAGH

The Photochemistry and Photometabolism of Bilirubin

Introduction

Complete assessment of the safety of phototherapy and formulation of effective guidelines for its use will be difficult until it is known how phototherapy works. This will require a complete understanding of the photometabolism of bilirubin in the neonate, which, in turn, will probably require detailed knowledge of the photochemistry of bilirubin.

In this paper I shall discuss the photochemistry of bilirubin in solution *in vitro* and some recently discovered thermal reactions of bilirubin. This will be followed by some preliminary results of our current studies on the photometabolism of bilirubin in the jaundiced Gunn rat. The paper will conclude with some comments on the mechanism and potential hazards of phototherapy.

In Vitro *Photochemistry of Bilirubin*

Bilirubin has a strong absorption band in the visible at 420–460 nm. Irradiation of bilirubin solutions with light within this wavelength region

This work was aided by a grant from the United Cerebral Palsy Research and Educational Foundation, by U.S. Public Health Service Grant AM–11275, and by generous support and gifts of equipment from the Duro-Test Corporation, North Bergen, New Jersey.

will cause excitation of ground-state bilirubin to excited-state bilirubin (denoted by the asterisk) as in Eq. (1).

$$\text{Bilirubin} \xrightarrow[\sim 450\text{ nm}]{h\nu} \text{Bilirubin}^* \quad (1)$$

$$\text{Bilirubin}^* \xrightarrow[-\text{Energy}]{} \text{Bilirubin} \quad (2)$$

$$\text{Bilirubin}^* \xrightarrow{HX} \text{Bilirubin}\cdot HX \text{ (adduct)} \quad (3)$$

$$\text{Bilirubin}^* \xrightarrow{O_2} \text{Oxidation products} \quad (4)$$

Following this primary event, the excited-state bilirubin can undergo three secondary processes, the process depending on the reaction conditions. These processes are as follows (see Addendum, p. 71):

Radiationless decay back to the ground state, Eq. (2). This is, of course, a trivial process.

Photoaddition, Eq. (3).

Photooxidation, Eq. (4).

PHOTOADDITION

Irradiation of bilirubin in the presence of alcohols or thiols results in Markovnikoff addition to the *exo*-vinyl group of the bilirubin molecule (Figure 1).[14–16] This reaction has been shown to occur with primary and secondary alcohols,[14] 2-mercaptoethanol,[15] glutathione,[16] and *N*-acetyl-L-cysteine.[16] So far, the reaction has only been observed to occur under anaerobic conditions; and relative to the well-known photooxidation of bilirubin that takes place under aerobic conditions, photoaddition appears to be a slow reaction.

Of particular interest with respect to the mechanism of phototherapy is Manitto's observation [14] that, when bilirubin is irradiated in chloroform in the absence of methanol under nitrogen and methanol is then added

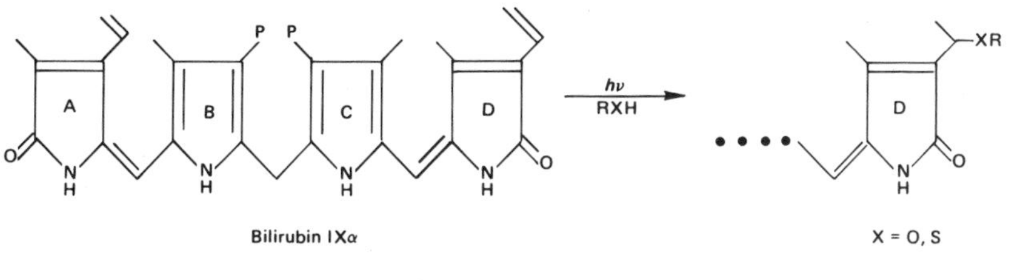

FIGURE 1 Diagram of photoaddition of alcohols and thiols to bilirubin.

to the solution in the dark, the methanol adduct ($XR=OCH_3$ in Figure 1) is still formed. This observation is intriguing because it indicates that irradiation of bilirubin can lead to an excited state or photoisomer having a lifetime of at least a few seconds.

PHOTOOXIDATION

When bilirubin is irradiated in the presence of air or oxygen, the pigment is photooxidized to a mixture of products containing biliverdin, propentdyopents, methylvinylmaleimide, hematinic acid imide, and unidentified other constituents.[2, 9–11] There is evidence that the photooxidation can proceed simultaneously via two main pathways (Figure 2).[3, 8, 18] One pathway (I) leads to biliverdin and then, by a very slow photochemical reaction, to lower molecular weight products. The other pathway (II) leads directly from bilirubin to mono- and dipyrrolic products. The relative importance of these two routes varies with the reaction conditions, especially the nature of the solvent and the initial bilirubin concentration. However, although *some* biliverdin is invariably formed when bilirubin is photooxidized, pathway II predominates under all *in vitro* conditions so far studied.

Therefore, biliverdin is not an intermediate in the main pathway of bilirubin photooxidation as formerly proposed.[26] It should be noted that biliverdin, unlike bilirubin, is relatively stable to photooxidation[3, 8, 18] and actually *inhibits* photooxidation of bilirubin.[18] As far as phototherapy is concerned, it is unlikely that formation of biliverdin makes any important contribution to the lowering of levels of serum bilirubin during irradiation *in vivo*. If any biliverdin were formed, it would surely be reduced back to bilirubin by the ubiquitous enzyme biliverdin reductase.[30]

Abundant evidence exists that photooxidation of bilirubin *in vitro* is predominantly a photochemical Type II process involving singlet oxygen (i.e., molecular oxygen in its first excited singlet energy state).[3, 19] In this process (Figure 3), absorption of light by ground-state bilirubin leads to formation of bilirubin in its first excited singlet state, which by

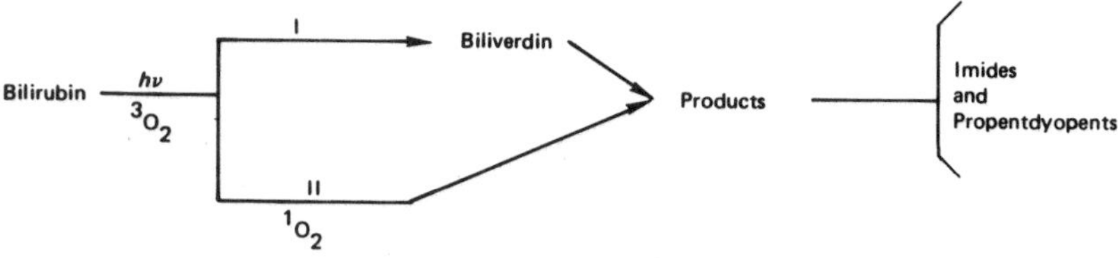

FIGURE 2 Diagram showing pathways for the photooxidation of bilirubin.

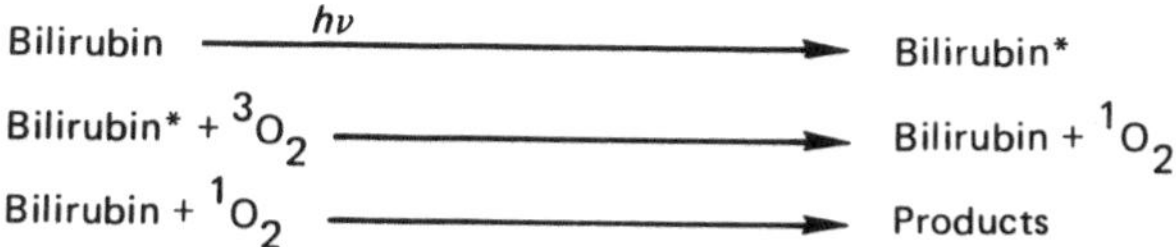

FIGURE 3 Diagram showing the mechanism of bilirubin photooxidation. (Asterisk indicates triplet excited state.)

intersystem crossover converts to triplet bilirubin. Triplet bilirubin interacts with ground-state (triplet) oxygen ($^3O_2$) to give ground-state bilirubin and singlet oxygen ($^1O_2$). Rapid attack of bilirubin by singlet oxygen then leads to products.

The evidence for the involvement of singlet oxygen in the reaction is as follows:

1. The rate of the reaction is accelerated by the presence of known singlet-oxygen sensitizers, such as porphyrins, methylene blue, or rose bengal,[19] with no qualitative difference in the nature of the photoproducts.[9]
2. The reaction is inhibited by singlet oxygen quenchers, such as β-carotene and certain tertiary amines.[3, 19] (The observed inhibition by biliverdin,[18] mentioned above, is due to quenching of singlet oxygen also by biliverdin.)
3. The reaction is competitively inhibited by compounds that react readily with singlet oxygen.[19]
4. Singlet oxygen can be "trapped" during the reaction by the addition of dimethyl furan, and the corresponding derivative of dimethyl furan has been isolated.[3]
5. The reaction is accelerated when it is carried out in certain deuterated solvents in which the lifetime of singlet oxygen is increased.[3]
6. The products that have been isolated from the photooxidation are those expected on the basis of a singlet-oxygen mechanism.[2, 9–11]

There is, therefore, convincing evidence that bilirubin is a photosensitizer and that the photooxidation of bilirubin *in vitro* is a self-sensitized reaction involving singlet oxygen. This finding explains why bilirubin has photodynamic properties and can cause photohemolysis of red cells *in vitro*.[6, 24, 27]

In vivo bilirubin is largely associated with albumin. The albumin molecule contains unsaturated amino acid residues that react with singlet oxygen [22, 29] and that, in the presence of bilirubin, could compete with

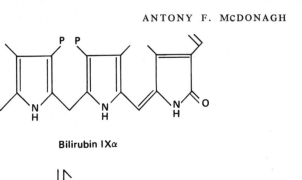

2

P P

O N H N H N H N H O

Bilirubin IXα

(Initiator) O_2

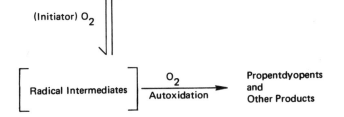

[Radical Intermediates] $\xrightarrow[\text{Autoxidation}]{O_2}$ Propentdyopents and Other Products

(Initiator) O_2

P P

O N H N H N H N H O

Bilirubin IIIα

+

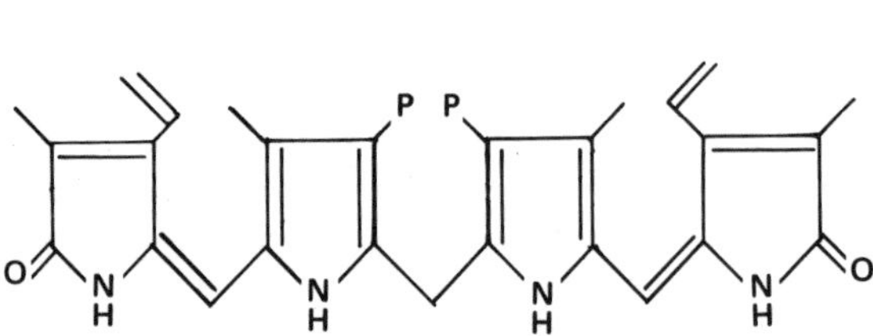

Bilirubin XIIIα

FIGURE 4 Diagram of the isomerization and autoxidation of bilirubin in water.

the pigment for singlet oxygen. Hence, the photooxidation of bilirubin in serum or in aqueous solutions containing albumin is likely to be slower than it would be in the absence of protein. Under these conditions, the Type I process (Figure 2) may assume greater importance.

Nonphotochemical Reactions of Bilirubin in Aqueous Media

Although bilirubin is relatively stable in the dark in organic solvents (e.g., chloroform, dimethyl sulfoxide, and ammoniacal methanol), it is not as stable in water, especially in the absence of binding proteins or stabilizers. This instability makes photochemical studies of bilirubin in water more complicated. Therefore, the dark reactions that bilirubin tends to undergo in aqueous solution are worth considering briefly.

Recent studies have shown that at least two major reactions, autooxidation and isomerization, occur simultaneously when bilirubin is dissolved in aqueous buffers within the pH range of about 7.4–12 (Ref. 20 and unpublished observations by A. F. McDonagh, F. Assisi, and L. Palma).

AUTOXIDATION

When aqueous solutions of bilirubin are exposed to air or oxygen in the dark, the pigment slowly disappears and is converted predominantly into colorless products. If the reaction is followed by spectrophotometry, a sequence of changes is observed that is qualitatively similar to the sequence observed when bilirubin is photooxidized. Although the products of the reaction have not been identified, they give a strong positive propentdyopent test, indicating that they may be similar to the photooxidation products of bilirubin. In the presence of albumin, this autoxidation reaction is markedly inhibited.

ISOMERIZATION

Under the same conditions, bilirubin not only autoxidizes but also isomerizes to a mixture containing three isomers: bilirubin IIIα, bilirubin IXα, and bilirubin XIIIα (Figure 4). This reaction is reversible and occurs readily at physiological pH and temperature.

The detailed mechanism of the isomerization reaction is not clear, but free radical intermediates appear to be involved, and, under normal conditions, it is atmospheric oxygen that initiates the process. In the absence of oxygen or other radical initiators, the reaction does not occur. The reaction is inhibited by radical scavengers, such as ascorbic acid and glutathione, and does not occur when the bilirubin is bound to albumin.

Therefore, in an aqueous solution of bilirubin in equilibrium with air at moderately basic pH values, two interrelated reactions are occurring.

There is a rapid and reversible isomerization of the bilirubin, and there is a slower bleeding-off of the pigment to autoxidation products. The relative importance of each reaction appears to vary with the oxygen tension and initial concentration of bilirubin. It is not clear whether either of these reactions has any direct relevance to phototherapy. However, the reactions should be taken into account in photochemical and toxicity studies of bilirubin done in aqueous solution. In addition, they may be involved in the alternative pathways of bilirubin metabolism,[28] which lead to bilirubin degradation products, and in the formation of the lower-molecular-weight products that are excreted during phototherapy. (See "Mechanism of Phototherapy," p. 67).

Photometabolism of Bilirubin

STUDIES ON PHOTOSENSITIZED GUNN RATS*

Singlet-oxygen sensitizers, including porphyrins, accelerate the photooxidation of bilirubin *in vitro.*[19] Since it is not known whether singlet oxygen is involved in the photodegradation of bilirubin *in vivo,* we have studied the effect of an exogenous singlet-oxygen sensitizer on the efficiency of phototherapy in the congenitally jaundiced Gunn rat.

As photosensitizer, we used commercial hematoporphyrin, treated according to the method of Lipson *et al.*[12] Apart from its phototoxicity, this material is nontoxic; it is water soluble and probably binds to albumin. Following intravenous injection into the Gunn rat (0.5 mg/100 g), the serum concentration of the drug remains high for the first few hours and within 24 h decreases to undetectable concentrations.

We have done two types of experiment. In the first (Figure 5), shaved and depilated rats were injected intravenously with vehicle (saline) and 1 h later exposed to visible light from a Vita-Lite fixture for 5 h. Following a recovery period of about 60 h, the rats were injected with a solution of hematoporphyrin and kept in the dark for almost 70 h. Finally, the rats were reinjected with hematoporphyrin and 1 h later re-exposed to the light for 5 h, and then kept in the dark for an additional 70 h. In the second type of experiment (Figure 6), three male Gunn rats of similar age and weight were shaved and depilated on their backs. One rat was injected with saline and two rats were injected with hematoporphyrin. After 1.5 h, the saline rat and one of the porphyrin-treated rats were exposed to visible light (Vita-Lite) for 4 h and then kept in the dark for 42 h. The other porphyrin-treated rat was kept in the dark throughout the experiment. During both types of experiment, tail-vein

* A. F. McDonagh, unpublished observations.

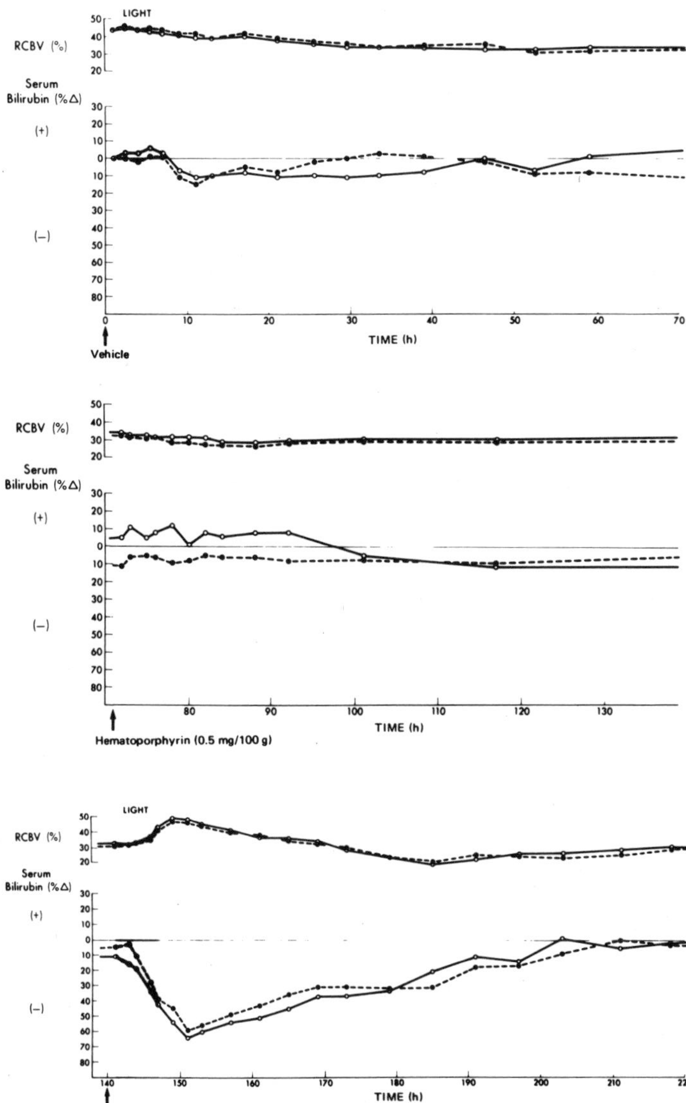

FIGURE 5 Effect of hematoporphyrin photosensitization on red blood cell volume and serum bilirubin concentration of Gunn rats during phototherapy (Vita-Lite, 600 ft-c). Data from two rats are plotted (broken line and solid line). The three graphs represent one continuous experiment. The rats were kept in darkness except during the two light periods, when they were exposed to light from a Vita-Lite fixture. *Top:* Effect of light. *Center:* Effect of hematoporphyrin. *Bottom:* Effect of hematoporphyrin and light.

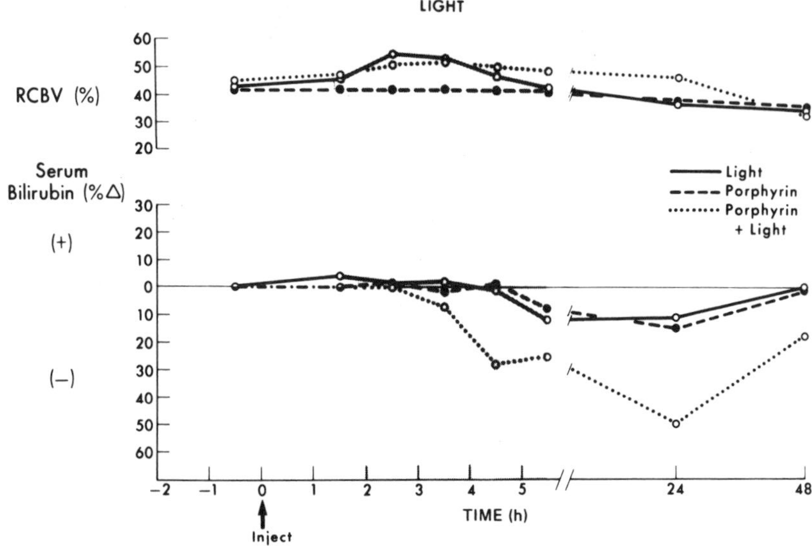

FIGURE 6 Effect of hematoporphyrin photosensitization on red blood cell volume and serum bilirubin concentration of the Gunn rat during exposure to light (Vita-Lite, 600 ft-c).

blood samples were collected periodically. These were used to determine red blood cell volumes and serum bilirubin concentrations (by the diazo method). The serum bilirubin concentration and red blood cell volume in the first blood sample drawn from each rat at the beginning of each experiment were arbitrarily taken as the norm for that rat, and subsequent values were expressed as a percentage change from the norm value.

The experimental results (Figures 5 and 6) show that there was no marked change in concentration of serum bilirubin when the rats were injected with saline and exposed to light. Nor was there any marked change when the rats were injected with porphyrin and kept in the dark. But when the animals were injected with porphyrin and then exposed to light, there was a rapid and pronounced drop in the concentration of serum bilirubin. The concentration continued to decrease for several hours after the light was turned off, and then gradually returned to normal. The observed fall in concentration was not an artifact caused by dilution of the serum with extravascular fluid, since red blood cell volumes did not decrease significantly while the bilirubin concentration was falling.

Therefore, treatment of a jaundiced animal with light *and* a photosensitizer can cause a much more rapid fall in concentration of serum bilirubin than treatment with light alone.

It is tempting to speculate that the effect of the photosensitizer is merely to speed up the processes that normally occur during phototherapy, perhaps by generating singlet oxygen and enhancing bilirubin photooxidation. Unfortunately we do not have sufficient data to support this hypothesis, and the alternative explanation that the fall in serum bilirubin is due to a shift of the pigment into extravascular tissue must be considered equally valid. However, the experiments do show that a singlet-oxygen sensitizer other than bilirubin can produce the desired phototherapeutic effect. The results also suggest that endogenous photosensitizers, such as naturally occurring porphyrins or riboflavin, could play a role in phototherapy.

PHOTOMETABOLISM OF BILIRUBIN IN THE GUNN RAT *

When jaundiced infants or Gunn rats are exposed to visible light, there is a change in the constitution of the bile and, eventually, a fall in concentration of serum bilirubin.[4, 25]

Isotope-labeling experiments using ^{14}C-bilirubin have shown that the light exposure causes a sharp increase in the excretion of radioactivity, particularly into the bile. This increase is due partly to enhanced excretion of bilirubin catabolites [4, 25] and partly to enhanced biliary excretion of unconjugated bilirubin.[25]

We recently started studying the photoproducts in the bile of the Gunn rat. Our aims are as follows:

- To confirm that there is increased output of bilirubin (as opposed to some closely related structural analogue) during phototherapy.
- To determine what proportion of the photoproducts this unconjugated bilirubin (or bilirubinoid fraction) accounts for.
- To identify the remaining nonbilirubinoid photoproducts.

In this section I shall discuss some *preliminary findings* related to the first two of these aims. For simplicity, results of a single experiment on a single rat will be presented; this is, however, a reproducible experiment.

A male homozygous Gunn rat was shaved on its back and residual hair was removed with a depilatory cream. The bile duct was cannulated and a catheter was introduced into the femoral vein for intravenous

* A. F. McDonagh, unpublished observations.

infusion. The animal, placed in a restraining cage with access to food and water, was continuously infused with isotonic saline–dextrose solution. The animal was injected intravenously with a pulse of ^{14}C-bilirubin ($t=0$) and kept in the dark for 12 h. Then bile was collected for three consecutive 4-hour periods in the dark, for three 4-hour periods with the animal exposed to light from a Vita-Lite fixture, and, finally, for three 4-hour periods with the animal again in the dark. All bile was collected on ice in the dark. At the end of each 4-hour period, each volume of bile was measured. Each sample was then vigorously stirred, examined visually for any signs of precipitate or turbidity, sampled for counting, and finally frozen and stored. The bile flow remained constant throughout the experiment. At the end of the experiment, bile samples were thawed, stirred, re-examined, and centrifuged. Samples of each supernatant were then taken for counting.

Figure 7 shows the changes observed periodically in the biliary excretion of radioactivity during the experiment. The results confirm the experience of previous investigators [4, 25] and show that exposure to light causes a large increase in biliary radioactivity that gradually diminishes following removal of the animal from the light source.

All the bile samples were clear, but samples collected during the light period were markedy pigmented. When the samples were thawed after having been frozen, an orange precipitate was observed in those collected during and just after the light period. In contrast, the pre-light bile samples remained clear. Following centrifugation and removal of the precipitate, there was a pronounced drop in the total counts of the on-light bile samples (Figure 8). The radioactivity of each orange precipitate was calculated from the difference in radioactivity of the corresponding bile sample before and after centrifugation. These data are plotted in Figure 9.

From Figures 8 and 9, it can be deduced (1) that the precipitable fraction accounts for about 60 percent of the total radioactivity excreted into the bile during the on-light period and (2) that about 70 percent of the *increase* in excreted radioactivity that occurs during the light period is contained in the precipitate.

We are investigating the nature of the orange precipitate. Although it has different solubility properties than bilirubin (e.g., it is not readily soluble in chloroform or 0.1 mol/l sodium hydroxide), it has a visible absorption spectrum identical to bilirubin IXα in dimethyl sulfoxide. By mild aqueous treatment of a solution of the precipitate in dimethyl sulfoxide, it is converted to bilirubin IXα. Therefore, the main constituent of the pigment has an intact bilirubin tetrapyrrole nucleus. The precipitate is probably a weak ionic complex or salt of bilirubin, perhaps calcium bilirubinate.

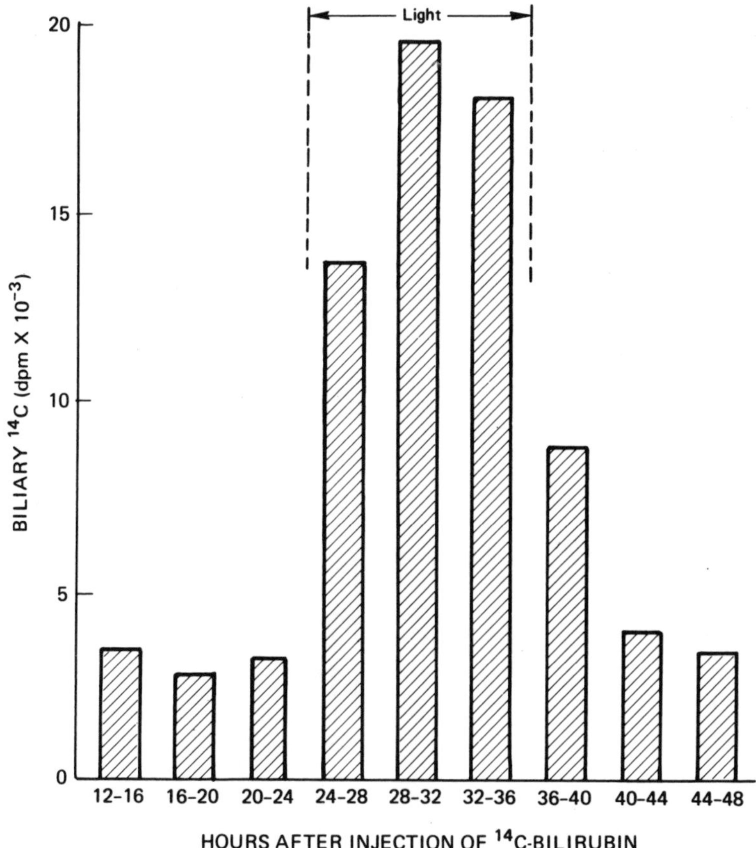

FIGURE 7 Effect of light (Vita-Lite, 800 ft-c) on the total biliary excretion of radioactivity in a Gunn rat labeled with ^{14}C-bilirubin.

In conclusion, it appears that the main effect of phototherapy in the Gunn rat is to enhance the output of either bilirubin or bilirubin anion. Therefore, the major pathway in phototherapy may *not* involve photo-oxidation or photodegradation of bilirubin; instead, it may involve enhanced excretion of bilirubin IXα. This finding is supported by recent studies of the effect of phototherapy on jaundiced babies.[13]

Mechanism of Phototherapy

The mechanism of phototherapy is still obscure. The vague outline that is beginning to emerge is shown in Figure 10. According to this scheme,

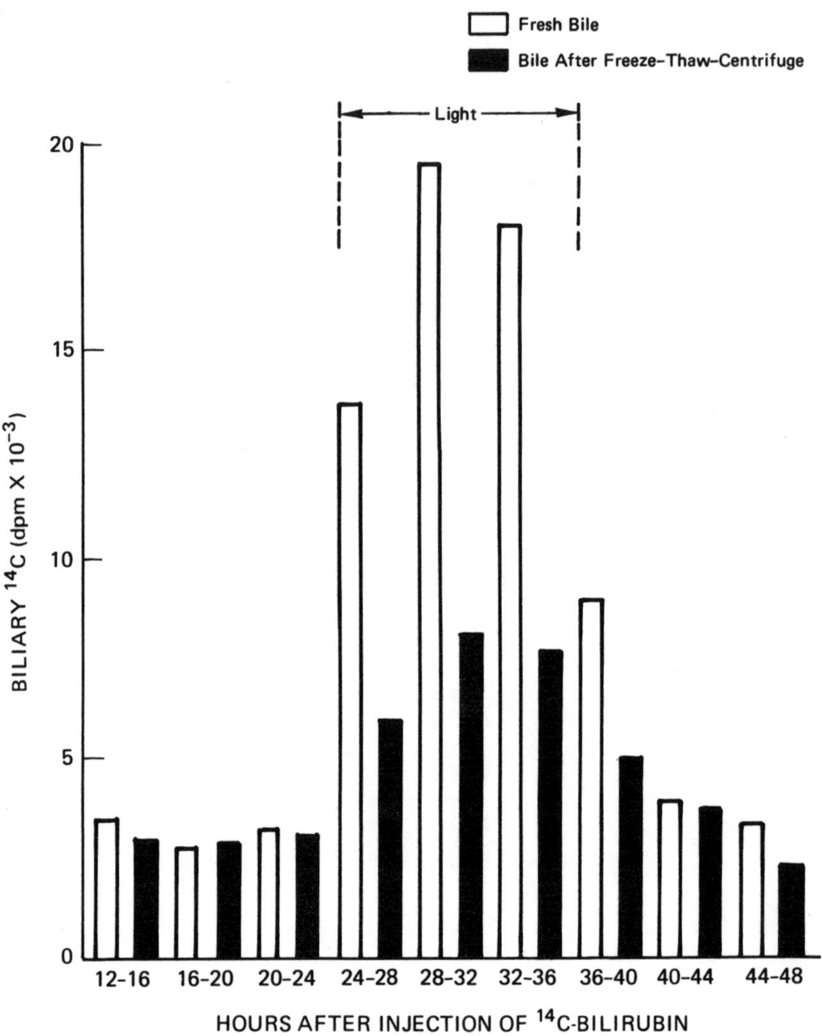

FIGURE 8 Total biliary radioactivity of bile from a labeled Gunn rat exposed to light before (open bars) and after (solid bars) removal of the precipitable fraction.

absorption of light by bilirubin leads to excited-state bilirubin. By some unknown mechanism, the bilirubin ultimately passes through the liver and into the bile. This mechanism appears to be the main pathway. Bilirubin derivatives of lower molecular weight could arise in at least two ways. Excited-state bilirubin in the tissue could interact with oxygen

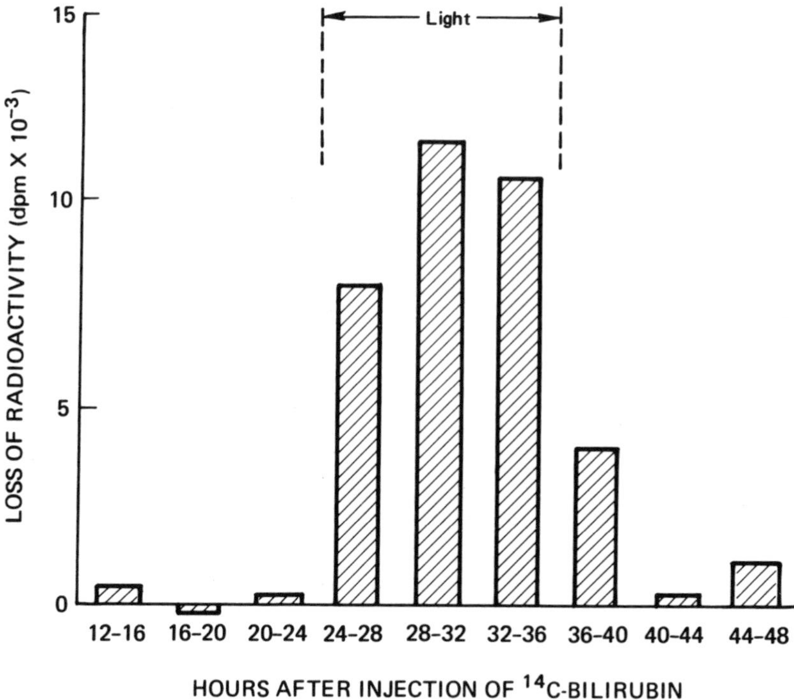

FIGURE 9 Total radioactivity of the precipitable fraction from the bile of a labeled Gunn rat exposed to light.

to give singlet oxygen, which could then attack the bilirubin to give readily excretable compounds of lower molecular weight. Alternatively, the bilirubin catabolites could arise by autoxidation of bilirubin by the reaction discussed under "Photometabolism of Bilirubin," p. 62.

Hazards of Phototherapy

Potential hazards of two types can be distinguished, those related to bilirubin and those not related. The latter include general biological effects of visible light on a variety of physiological functions and photodynamic effects of endogenous photosensitizers other than bilirubin; these will not be discussed here. The main bilirubin-related hazards are photoproduct toxicity and photodynamic damage.

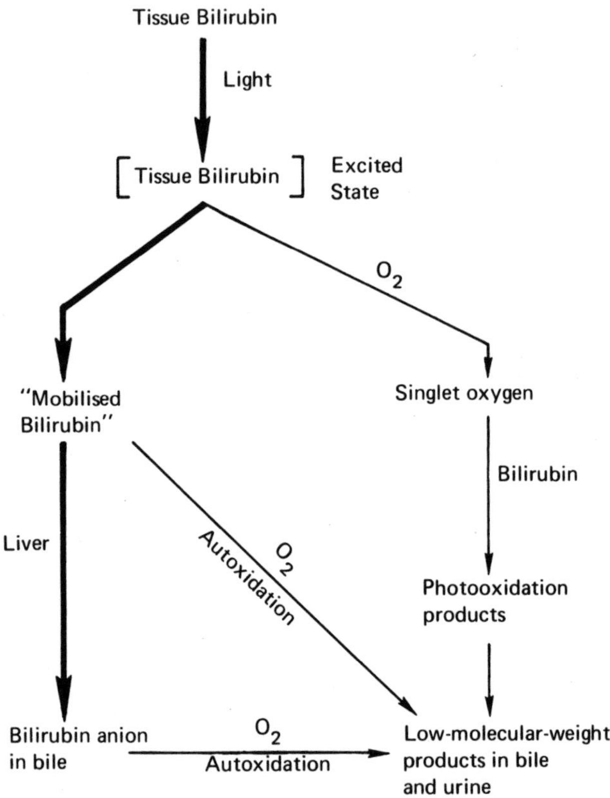

FIGURE 10 Schematic outline of the mechanism of phototherapy.

PHOTOPRODUCT TOXICITY

If indeed the main "photoproduct" is unconjugated bilirubin itself (i.e., enhanced biliary excretion of bilirubin), photoproduct toxicity is not likely to be a serious hazard. However, until all the photoproducts have been identified and tested pharmacologically, this hazard cannot be completely evaluated.

PHOTODYNAMIC DAMAGE

Bilirubin is a photosensitizer.[6, 19, 24, 27] In this respect, it is similar to porphyrins, chlorophylls, and other photodynamic agents. However, it differs from these other photosensitizers in two important ways.[19] First, it is an inefficient photosensitizer. Second, it is itself readily attacked and destroyed by singlet oxygen. For these reasons, bilirubin, unlike porphyrins and chlorophyll, is not a powerful photodynamic agent. This fits with common experience. When exposed to sunlight, jaundiced people of all ages and those with bilirubin-pigmented bruises do not develop any of the characteristic symptoms that result from photodynamic damage. Therefore, gross photodynamic damage can be ruled out as a major hazard of phototherapy.

Nevertheless, minor, more subtle, photodynamic effects could occur during phototherapy, and we should consider what these might be and whether they may have serious consequences.

Since bilirubin is predominantly bound to albumin *in vivo,* and since singlet oxygen (which is believed to cause photodynamic damage)[5, 7, 22] has a very brief lifetime in solution,[17, 21] the main loci for photodynamic damage are likely to be residues of unsaturated amino acids in the albumin molecule. Damage to other tissue constituents is less likely because albumin, by competing with bilirubin for singlet oxygen, should shield neighboring molecules from bilirubin-sensitized attack.

At present there is no evidence, either from *in vitro* or *in vivo* experiments, to indicate that significant photosensitized oxygenation of albumin occurs during phototherapy. Since photosensitized oxidation of albumin reduces its bilirubin-binding capacity,[23] which might in turn increase the risk of kernicterus,[23] this aspect of phototherapy merits investigation.

In vitro, bilirubin can cause photodynamic hemolysis of erythrocytes,[6, 24, 27] and it has been suggested that photohemolysis may occur during phototherapy. At the light intensities commonly used for phototherapy, this is unlikely to be significant *in vivo* for three reasons: (1) bilirubin is a weak photosensitizer; (2) serum bilirubin is albumin-bound and, as discussed above, the albumin will exert a protective effect; and (3) light absorption by oxyhemoglobin will markedly reduce the intensity of photodynamically active light ($\sim$450 nm) reaching the bilirubin. In agreement with this, there is no clinical evidence that photohemolysis occurs during phototherapy.[1]

In summary, there do not appear to be any deleterious effects of phototherapy associated with the interaction of bilirubin and light. Although this seems reassuring, it is too soon to be complacent.

Addendum

Since this paper was presented, we have discovered two novel photochemical reactions of bilirubin that are mentioned here for the sake of completeness.

1. Irradiation of bilirubin IXα in aqueous solution at pH 8.5 with visible light in the *absence of oxygen* leads to formation of bilirubin IIIα and bilirubin XIIIα (Figure 4). In the presence of albumin or in organic solvents, this reaction does not occur and isomers are not formed. This finding provides additional evidence that a radical process is involved in the isomerization of bilirubin that occurs in the presence of oxygen in the dark.

2. Irradiation of bilirubin IXα at pH 8.5 in aqueous solution with visible light in the presence of serum albumin and the *absence of oxygen* leads to formation of a yellow photoderivative (λ_{max} 442–444 nm in chloroform). This compound is slightly more polar and less lipophilic than bilirubin at slightly basic pH values. Its identity and properties are being investigated.

REFERENCES

1. Blackburn, M. G., and M. M. Orzalesi. Effect of light on fetal red blood cells in vitro, p. 265. The American Pediatric Society, Inc. and the Society for Pediatric Research. Combined Program and Abstracts, Traymore Hotel, Atlantic City, New Jersey, April 28–May 1, 1971. (A)
2. Bonnett, R., and J. C. M. Stewart. Photo-oxidation of bilirubin in hydroxylic solvents: Propentdyopent adducts as major products. J.C.S. Chem. Commun. 596–597, 1972.
3. Bonnett, R., and J. C. M. Stewart. Singlet oxygen in the photo-oxidation of bilirubin in hydroxylic solvents. Biochem. J. 130:895–897, 1972.
4. Callahan, E. W., Jr., M. M. Thaler, M. Karon, K. Bauer, and R. Schmid. Phototherapy of severe unconjugated hyperbilirubinemia: Formation and removal of labeled bilirubin derivatives. Pediatrics 46:841–848, 1970.
5. Foote, C. S., and R. W. Denny. Chemistry of singlet oxygen. VII. Quenching by β-carotene. (communication to the editor) J. Am. Chem. Soc. 90:6233–6235, 1968.
6. Hausmann, W. Ueber die sensibilisierende Wirkung tierischer Farbstoffe und ihre physiologische Bedeutung. Biochem. Z. 4:275–278, 1908.
7. Kearns, D. R. Physical and chemical properties of singlet molecular oxygen. Chem. Rev. 71:395–427, 1971.
8. Lightner, D. A., D. C. Crandall, S. Gertler, and G. B. Quistad. On the formation of biliverdin during photooxygenation of bilirubin *in vitro*. FEBS Lett. 30:309–312, 1973.
9. Lightner, D. A., and G. B. Quistad. Hematinic acid and propentdyopents from bilirubin photo-oxidation *in vitro*. FEBS Lett. 25:94–96, 1972.
10. Lightner, D. A., and G. B. Quistad. Imide products from photo-oxidation of bilirubin and mesobilirubin. Nature (New Biol.) 236:203–205, 1972.
11. Lightner, D. A., and G. B. Quistad. Methylvinylmaleimide from bilirubin photooxidation. Science 175:324, 1972.
12. Lipson, R. L., E. J. Baldes, and A. M. Olsen. The use of a derivative of hematoporphyrin in tumor detection. J. Natl. Cancer Inst. 26:1–11, 1961.

13. Lund, H. T., and J. Jacobsen. Influence of phototherapy on unconjugated bilirubin in duodenal bile of newborn infants with hyperbilirubinemia. A preliminary study. Acta Paediatr. Scand. 61:693–696, 1972.
14. Manitto, P. Photochemistry of bilirubin. Experientia 27:1147–1149, 1971.
15. Manitto, P., and D. Monti. Photoaddition of sulphydryl groups to bilirubin *in vitro*. Experientia 28:379–380, 1972.
16. Manitto, P., D. Monti, and E. Garbagnati. Photochemical addition of *N*-acetyl-L-cysteine and glutathione to bilirubin *in vitro* and its relevance to phototherapy of jaundice. Farmaco 27:999–1002, 1972.
17. Matheson, I. B. C., and J. Lee. Lifetime of ($^1\Delta_g$) oxygen in solution. Chem. Phys. Lett. 14:350–351, 1972.
18. McDonagh, A. F. Evidence for singlet oxygen quenching by biliverdin IX-α dimethyl ester and its relevance to bilirubin photo-oxidation. Biochem. Biophys. Res. Commun. 48:408–415, 1972.
19. McDonagh, A. F. The role of singlet oxygen in bilirubin photo-oxidation. Biochem. Biophys. Res. Commun. 44:1306–1311, 1971.
20. McDonagh, A. F., and F. Assisi. The ready isomerization of bilirubin IX-α in aqueous solution. Biochem. J. 129:797–800, 1972.
21. Merkel, P. B., and D. R. Kearns. Remarkable solvent effects on the lifetime of $^1\Delta_g$ oxygen. (Communication to the editor) J. Am. Chem. Soc. 94:1029–1030, 1972.
22. Nilsson, R., P. B. Merkel, and D. R. Kearns. Unambiguous evidence for the participation of singlet oxygen (1) in photodynamic oxidation of amino acids. Photochem. Photobiol. 16:117–124, 1972.
23. Odell, G. B., R. S. Brown, and N. A. Holtzman. Dye-sensitized photo-oxidation of albumin associated with a decreased capacity for protein-binding of bilirubin. Birth Defects 6:31–35, 1970.
24. Odell, G. B., R. S. Brown, and A. E. Kopelman. The photodynamic action of bilirubin on erythrocytes. J. Pediatr. 81:473–483, 1972.
25. Ostrow, J. D. Photocatabolism of labeled bilirubin in the congenitally jaundiced (Gunn) rat. J. Clin. Invest. 50:707–718, 1971.
26. Ostrow, J. D., and R. V. Branham. Photodecomposition of bilirubin and biliverdin *in vitro*. Gastroenterology 58:15–25, 1970.
27. Saeki, K. Studies in photodynamic haemolytic action of bilirubin; presence or absence of photodynamic haemolytic action, inquiry into factors concerned in it, after-effects of action and presence or absence of photodynamic haemolytic action in biliverdin. Jap. J. Gastroenterol. 4:153–165, 1932.
28. Schmid, R. Hyperbilirubinemia, pp. 1141–1178. In J. B. Stanbury, J. B. Wyngaarden, and D. S. Fredrickson, Eds. The Metabolic Basis of Inherited Disease. (3rd ed.) New York: McGraw-Hill, Inc., 1972.
29. Spikes, J. D., and R. Straight. Sensitized photochemical processes in biological systems. Ann. Rev. Phys. Chem. 18:409–436, 1967.
30. Tenhunen, R., M. E. Ross, H. S. Marver, and R. Schmid. Reduced nicotinamide–adenine dinucleotide phosphate dependent biliverdin reductase: Partial purification and characterization. Biochemistry 9:298–303, 1970.

J. DONALD OSTROW, COLIN S. BERRY, *and* JOHN E. ZAREMBO

Studies on the Mechanism of Phototherapy in the Congenitally Jaundiced Rat

Doctors Foote, Lightner, and McDonagh have beautifully elucidated the processes of photodegradation of bilirubin in the test tube (pp. 21, 34, and 56, this volume). However, the products that they have obtained *in vitro* are not the same as the photoderivatives that appear in the bile during phototherapy of the Gunn rat.[29] Therefore, it may not be valid to draw conclusions concerning the mechanisms of phototherapy *in vivo,* or the toxicity of the photoproducts, from results obtained with *in vitro* derivatives.[9, 15, 20, 38, 39]

It is not known whether different primary photoreactions occur *in vitro* and *in vivo,* or whether the same products are initially produced in both circumstances, but those formed *in vivo* are subsequently altered during their passage through the liver. However, since the initial photoproducts formed *in vivo* appear to be rapidly cleared and excreted in the bile,[28] only the derivatives found in the bile are available in sufficient quantity to permit study of their properties, such as toxicity, protein-binding, and distribution in the body.

Presented in part at the annual meetings of the American Association for the Study of Liver Diseases, Chicago, Illinois, November 1971 and 1972.[30, 31] This work was supported by research grants AM–14543 from the National Institutes of Health, U.S. Public Health Service, and MRIS 6680 from the U.S. Veterans Administration.

I will summarize studies that we have performed concerning the mechanism of phototherapy *in vivo,* studies in which the congenitally jaundiced homozygous Gunn rat was used as a model. Admittedly, the adult Gunn rat differs from the newborn human infant in respects other than species and age. One difference is that the adult Gunn rat has no capacity to conjugate bilirubin,[35] whereas the human neonate has some.[24] Another is that the neonatal primate has defective hepatic uptake of bilirubin [23] and defective biliary excretion of conjugated bilirubin,[7] whereas the Gunn rat is normal in these respects.[4, 6] Moreover, the Gunn rats in our experiments are provided with a biliary fistula, which interrupts the enterohepatic circulation. For these reasons, the results of our studies may not be entirely applicable to phototherapy of the human neonate.

Figure 1 shows a previously published experiment [28] on the effect of phototherapy on the biliary excretion of radioactive pigments by Gunn rats whose endogenous bilirubin pool had been labeled with tracer ^{14}C-bilirubin.[32] When the animals were exposed to intense illumination for 16 h (1600 ft-c), the excretion of ^{14}C was about 5 times greater than it was during the control period with the rats under dim light. Similar but less striking results were obtained with 500 ft-c of exposure, which is the usual therapeutic illumination for jaundiced infants. The output of diazo-

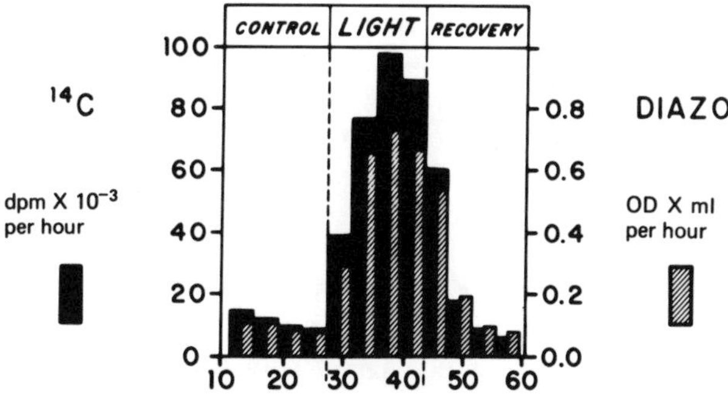

FIGURE 1 Effect of phototherapy on excretion rates of labeled bilirubin derivatives and diazo-reactive compounds in Gunn rat bile. A 350-gram rat was given 5 μCi ^{14}C-bilirubin intravenously at time 0 h, and bile collected in 4–hour aliquots thereafter. Control and recovery periods, 20 ft-c; light period, 1600 ft-c exposure from GE Daylite fluorescent lamps. (From Ostrow.[28])

reactive compounds [26] also increased, although less markedly, which indicated that some of the photoderivatives appearing in the bile were either not diazo-reactive or were less diazo-reactive than the ^{14}C-bilirubin from which they were derived. With the lights again extinguished during the recovery period, excretion of radioactivity and diazo-reactivity gradually declined to baseline values over the subsequent 8h, indicating that the processes involved were reversible.

Chromatography of the bile pigments, or of their ethyl anthranilate azopigments, revealed that most of the diazo-reactive material excreted during phototherapy was unconjugated bilirubin.[28] As a result of this experiment, two mechanisms were postulated for the action of phototherapy: [28] (1) Bilirubin is converted to polar photoderivatives that can be excreted in the bile without glucuronide conjugation; (2) the excretion of unconjugated bilirubin in bile is markedly augmented. Other experiments concerned the nature of these two mechanisms.

What Are the Polar Derivatives in the Bile?

McDonagh has clearly documented that singlet oxygen is involved in the photoreactions of bilirubin in the test tube [25] and has presented evidence that this is also true *in vivo* (pp. 56, this volume). He predicted that two types of products would be formed by singlet-oxygen attack on either the vinyl or bridge double bonds of bilirubin,[25] but he did not isolate and identify these products. The 5,5′-diformyldipyrrylmethane that he postulated has been produced by the alkaline degradation of bilirubin in the dark,[34] but it has yet to be identified as a photoproduct of bilirubin in any system, either *in vitro* or *in vivo*.

To determine the *in vivo* photoproducts, we repeated the experiment shown in Figure 1, using two Gunn rats with bile fistulae. After 10 h for equilibration of the injected tracer, ^{14}C-bilirubin, the pale-yellow bile excreted under dim light was collected for 21 h (dark bile). The rats were then exposed to light for 21 h; after this exposure they yielded bile that was deeply yellow-brown and contained 3-times as much radioactivity (light bile). The two bile samples were separately subjected to a modified Folch solvent-partition at pH 7 [33] and then, at pH 3, to extraction of the upper phase with chloroform. Each of the extracts was analyzed for diazo-reactivity [26] and radioactivity, and then processed by thin-layer chromatography (TLC) to separate the bilirubin derivatives. Recoveries exceeded 92 percent of the initial radioactivity in the bile samples.

Distribution of radioactivity in the two phases of the Folch partition is shown in Figure 2 (left). Both the lower (organic) and upper (aqueous) phases from light bile contained more radioactivity than the corresponding phases from control bile, indicating that photoproducts had partitioned into both phases. However, much more of the additional radioactivity excreted during phototherapy appeared in the lower phase (F-fraction). This fraction was taken to dryness by flash evaporation at 50 °C, and the solid residue was washed with methanol to extract the photoproducts. As illustrated in Figure 2 (right), most of the labeled material in this phase from light bile was methanol-insoluble and proved to be predominantly unconjugated bilirubin. This identification was confirmed by absorption spectroscopy, oxidation to biliverdin, production of typical azopigments, comigration with pure bilirubin in multiple TLC systems, and mass spectroscopy. In contrast, the Gunn rat bile excreted in the dark contained only a trace of bilirubin.

The Folch upper phase, which had been freed of cholesterol and phospholipid by the initial partition, contained mainly bile pigments and bile salts. This phase was adjusted to pH 3 with 1*N* HCl and then extracted with chloroform. As shown in Figure 3, the radioactivity from dark bile partitioned almost equally into the two phases, whereas the

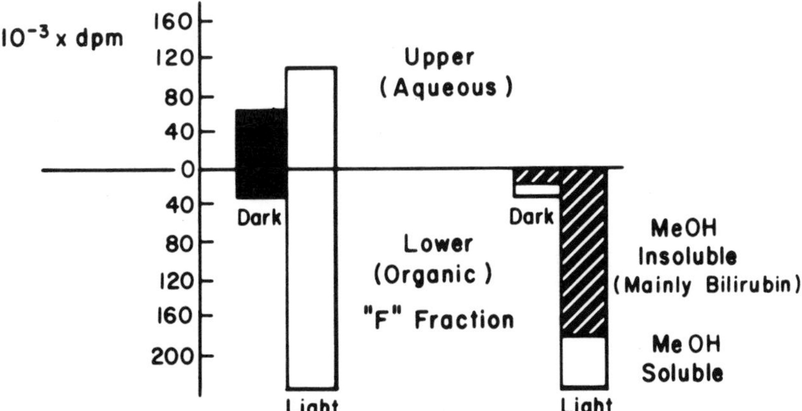

FIGURE 2 Distribution of radioactivity in the two phases of the Folch solvent-partition at pH 7 of pooled bile obtained from two Gunn rats each previously given 0.7 μCi of ^{14}C-bilirubin intravenously. Dark bile was collected from 12 to 33 h after administration of labeled bilirubin with animal under 20 ft-c illumination; light bile was collected from 33 to 54 h with the rat under 1600 ft-c illumination. Radioactivity in each phase referred to the total amount of labeled material excreted during each 21-hour collection period. Bars on the right refer to the soluble and insoluble fractions obtained by flash evaporation to dryness of the lower phase (F-fraction) and then extraction of the dried residue with methanol.

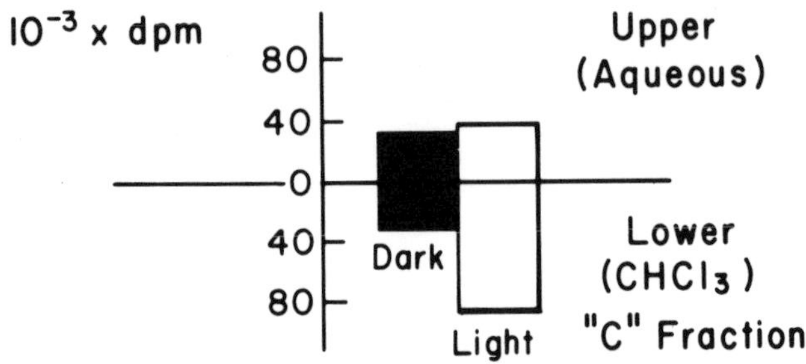

FIGURE 3 Radioactivity in the two phases obtained by chloroform extraction of the Folch upper phases from Figure 2, after acidification to pH 3.

radioactivity from light bile extracted principally into the chloroform, with almost no increase in the aqueous phase radioactivity due to phototherapy. Thus, almost all the ^{14}C-bilirubin photoderivatives were recovered in the chloroform phase at pH 3 (C-fraction). This suggested that the major photoproducts were anionic compounds with pK values between 3 and 7, typical of carboxyl groups. The pigments remaining in the aqueous fraction have not been identified, but they include almost half of the bilirubin metabolites excreted by the Gunn rat not exposed to phototherapy. This phase also contains all the bile salts, which in the rat are solely taurine conjugates.[21]

To summarize, the Folch extraction at pH 7 removed most of the bilirubin, while most of the photoderivatives were recovered at pH 3, in the chloroform extract, free of bile salts, cholesterol, and phospholipid. This C-fraction was subjected to TLC on silica gel, and each band was then eluted with chloroform–methanol and subjected to radioassay. As shown in Figure 4, 14 bands were obtained, which were designated in order of decreasing R_f. The horizontal axis represents the total radioactivity detected in each pigment band in the dark and in the light, respectively.

The pigments could be classified into three groups. Pigment C-9, which was pentdyopent-positive and therefore presumably a dipyrrole, was virtually undetectable in the dark but became the dominant pigment in light bile. A second group, best represented by C-5, was present in the dark bile but increased strikingly during phototherapy. A third group, represented by C-3 and C-10, was present in approximately equal quantities in dark and light bile and was therefore unrelated to phototherapy. Let me emphasize that all these separations were performed under very dim

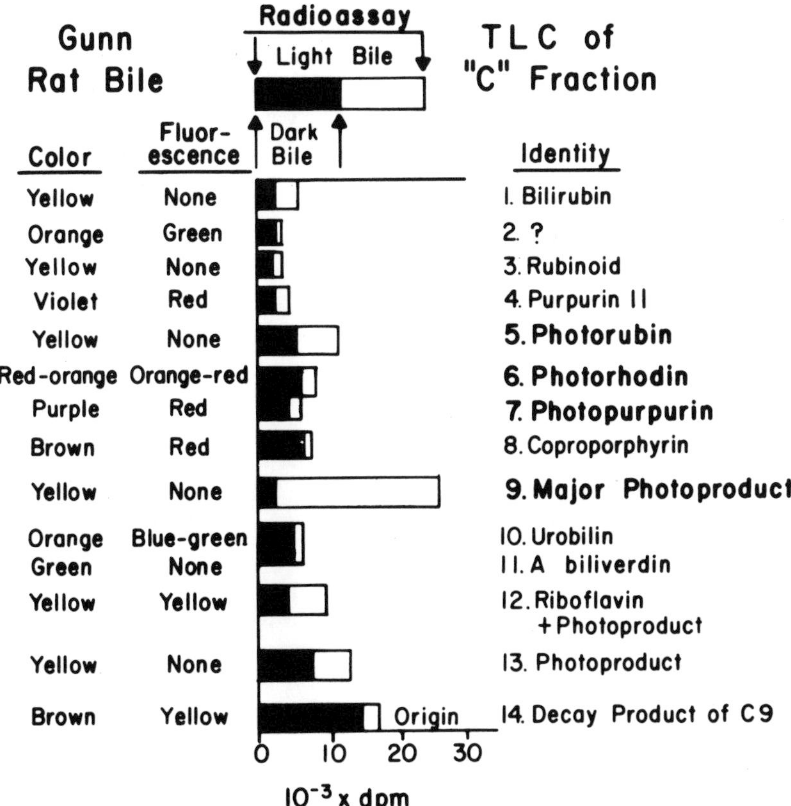

FIGURE 4 Representation of thin-layer chromatogram of C-fractions from Figure 3. Ascending chromatography performed for 75 min on 0.6-mm-thick layers of Camag silica gel D-5, with chloroform, methanol, and formic acid (30:3:1 by volume) as the developing solvent. Total excreted radioactivity in each eluted band from the dark and light biles is represented by the total height above the vertical baseline of the dark and light bars, respectively. Over 85 percent of the applied radioactivity was recovered in the eluted samples.

light; hence, the photoproducts that were found are not artifacts from *in vitro* photoreactions.

To obtain enough of these materials for identification requires huge volumes of Gunn rat bile. Therefore, it seemed worthwhile to again attempt to reproduce these products in the test tube, despite prior failures. A helpful clue was provided by the observation that jaundice disappears most rapidly from the exposed area of an infant's skin,[12] suggesting that the skin, and not the plasma, is the main site of bilirubin photodegradation *in vivo*. Since most of the bilirubin in Gunn rat skin is in the subcutaneous tissue,[36] we surmised that photodegradation might be occurring in a lipid, rather than an aqueous, environment, and that we could produce products *in vitro* that were identical to the photoproducts obtained *in vivo* if we simulated a lipid environment. Therefore, we dissolved bilirubin (20 mg/dl) in chloroform that had been washed previously with thiosulfate and then distilled to remove acidic impurities and the ethanol stabilizer. Photoderivatives were then prepared by exposing this solution to a 100-watt mercury spot lamp with a plate of glass interposed to reduce ultraviolet radiation.[8] The solution was mixed, oxygenated, and cooled by bubbling through it a stream of air. In 60 min, when 25 percent of the diazo-reactivity had disappeared, the solution was flash-evaporated to dryness and the residue was washed with methanol to extract the soluble photoproducts (Ch-fraction), which were then chromatographed as in Figure 4, alongside the C-fraction from Gunn rat bile.[8] Three spots were found that were present in both the *in vitro* and *in vivo* solutions: a nonfluorescent yellow spot that was also diazo positive (C-5/Ch-8), a red-orange spot with a pink to orange fluorescence (C-6/Ch-9), and a purple spot with a reddish fluorescence (C-7/Ch-10). None of the other spots in the two systems showed concordance. Methylvinylmaleimide (Ch-3) was isolated from the chloroform system but was not found in the Gunn rat bile, which is contrary to what one would expect if McDonagh's scheme for bilirubin photodegradation [25] applied to the *in vivo* system. C-12 in the Gunn bile was the strikingly yellow fluorescent material that Garay *et al.*[17] thought was the main bilirubin derivative excreted by the Gunn rat. On isolation, however, it proved to be riboflavin. The radioactivity present in this band was due to an overlapping photoproduct that was neither yellow nor yellow fluorescent. Compound C-2 resembled riboflavin in appearance, but it was much less polar and may be flavin with the ribose removed, or possibly lumichrome or lumiflavin.

The identity of the three products, which were found in both Gunn rat bile and the chloroform photoproducts, was further supported by correspondence of their R_f values in three other TLC systems and by correspondence of their methyl esters in two TLC solvent systems.[8] After purification through second- and third-stage TLC,[8] the corresponding products displayed identical absorption maxima, both as the native pigments and as their zinc complexes, and also yielded identical diazo derivatives and ferric chloride-oxidation products.[8] It therefore seemed reasonable to assume that the two groups of products were identical. They were further identified by mass spectrometric analysis of their methyl and trimethylsilyl (TMS) derivatives. Interpretation of the mass spectra was complicated by thermal degradation of the compounds in the insertion probe, presumably due to the large size and relatively polar nature of the photoproducts, which rendered them poorly volatile. Major ions obtained came from fragment ions, some of which also underwent subsequent dehydration.

C-5/Ch-8 was yellow, had a sharp absorption maximum at 422 nm, and formed a typical azopigment with an absorption maximum at 540 nm, like azobilirubin. However, the ratio of the optical density of azopigment at 540 nm to the optical density of the native pigment at its absorption maximum was only one fourth as great as would be found if the pigment had been bilirubin. Oxidation with 20-percent ferric chloride in concentrated hydrochloric acid at 80 °C yielded a green biliverdin product. These data indicated that C-5/Ch-8 was a tetrapyrrole with a bilirubin chromophore but possessed added polar groups on the middle single-bonded bridge that were inhibiting the diazo-reactivity of the molecule.

These conclusions from the chemical and spectral data were confirmed by the mass spectrometric data (Figure 5). The postulated structure of C-5/Ch-8 as a dihydroxybilirubin is shown in the figure as its dimethyl

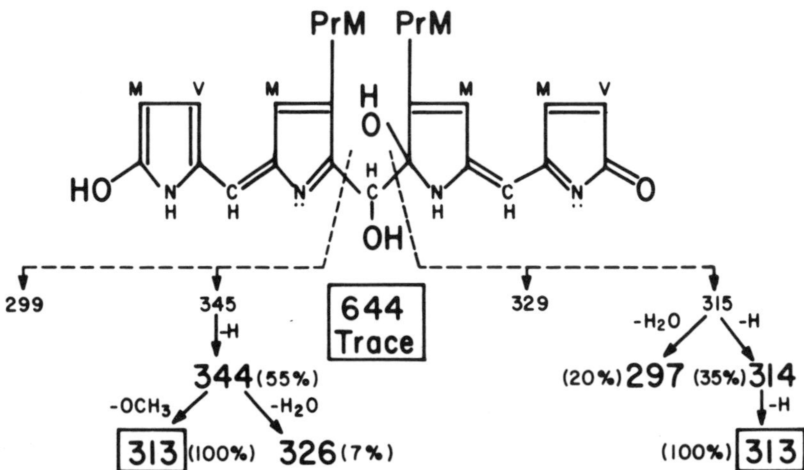

FIGURE 5 Proposed structural formula of the dimethyl ester of Gunn bile pigment C-5 (chloroform photoproduct Ch-8) with a rubin chromophore, showing fragmentation pattern accounting for the major ions obtained during mass spectroscopy. Large numbers are the *m/e* values of the major ions found; figures in parentheses represent the intensity of each ion as a percentage of the intensity of the base peak at $m/e = 313$. M = methyl, V = vinyl, Pr = propionic side-chains. Only one of two side-chain isomers is illustrated.

ester. The major ions obtained result from splits on either side of the hydroxylated bridge carbon, followed by loss of hydrogen or water from the resultant dipyrrole fragments. The base peak at $m/e=313$ could also result from loss of a methoxy group from the $m/e=344$ fragment ion. A trace of the molecular ion at $m/e=644$ was also found. The TMS derivative of the methyl ester yielded a molecular ion at $m/e=860$, indicating the addition of a TMS group to each of three hydroxyl groups in the molecule. The TMS derivative of the free acid showed large ions at $m/e=546$, 443, and 429, confirming the proposed arrangement of hydroxyl groups in the fragment ions of the parent molecule. The postulated structure is compatible with the one-fourth intensity of the diazo reaction of C-5/Ch-8. The diazo reagent would not couple with the right half-molecule because of the hydroxyl group on the pyrrole ring, and coupling of the left half-molecule would be retarded by steric hindrance from the two hydroxyl groups near the middle bridge.

C-6/Ch-9 had the characteristics of a rhodin chromophore, with a blood-red color and absorption maxima at 490, 328, and 265 nm. It was diazo negative, but its tetrapyrrole structure was confirmed by the formation of a verdin and a purpurin II on oxidation with ferric chloride. The zinc complex salt was blue with a brilliant orange-red fluorescence. Mass spectroscopy confirmed the structure shown in Figure 6, with a trace of molecular ion at $m/e=644$ and the base peak at $m/e=493$. Ions at $m/e=753$, 681, and 609 from the TMS derivative of the free acid, and at 637 and 565 from the TMS derivative of the dimethyl ester, confirmed

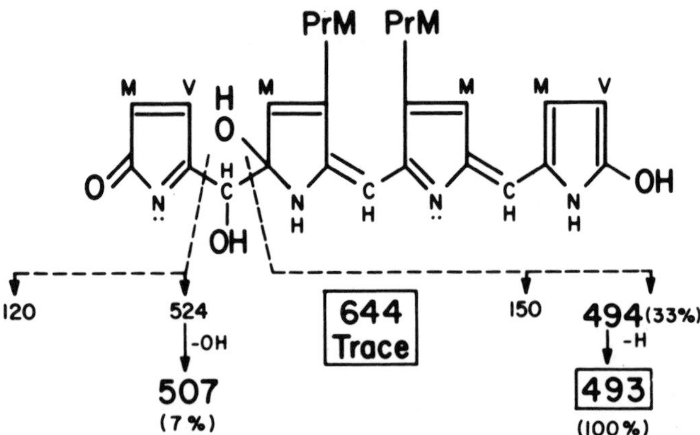

FIGURE 6 Proposed structural formula of the dimethyl ester of Gunn bile pigment C-6 (chloroform photoproduct Ch-9) with a rhodin chromophore, showing fragmentation pattern on mass spectroscopy, represented as in Figure 5.

the 493 ion from the dimethyl ester. A clear ion at $m/e = 578$ in the TMS derivative of the methyl ester confirmed the 507 fragment ion from the methyl ester and indicated that the left-hand hydroxyl group was attached to the bridge carbon rather than to the vinyl side-chain of the left-hand ring.

The third derivative, C-7/Ch-10, had the spectrochemical properties of a classic purpurin [37] with hydroxyl groups on the bridge carbon and on the adjacent α-carbon of the left-hand pyrrole ring. Its mass spectra have been difficult to interpret, so we cannot be sure of this structure.

We obtained two isomers of each of the three products and presume that these represent dihydroxyl additions to either the right- or left-hand portion of the bilirubin molecule, but we have not performed the nuclear magnetic resonance studies necessary to determine the disposition of side-chains in each isomer. We believe that these photoproducts derive from a singlet-oxygen mechanism because we observed a fourfold acceleration of the photoreaction on addition of methylene blue to the chloroform solution. To derive the products that were identified, one must postulate that light induces the formation of a high-energy phototautomer of bilirubin with a double–double–single bond arrangement of the bridges (Figure 7). Singlet oxygen could then add to either of the double bonds adjacent to the pyrrole ring second from the left, yielding the two photooxides or dioxetanes shown. Conversion to the dihydroxy derivatives would then involve transfer of hydrogens from one of the saturated bridges in the dioxetane.

This proposed mechanism is interesting for two reasons. First, the postulated phototautomer has a rhodin configuration and could thus represent the transient intermediate with an absorption maximum at 490 nm, which Davies and Keohane detected by using differential spectroscopy of irradiated bilirubin solutions.[13] Second, spatial considerations suggest that the intramolecular hydrogen transfer that converts the dioxetane into the dihydroxy derivatives could occur only if the intermediate had a cyclic porphyrinlike configuration. This configuration might account for the secondary peak at 410 nm, which was found in the action spectrum for photooxidation of bilirubin.[18] Of course, another possibility is that the planar bilirubin molecules are stacked and that the hydrogen transfer occurs inter- rather than intramolecularly.

We have thus identified for the first time several of the bilirubin derivatives formed during phototherapy of the jaundiced Gunn rat. It is fascinating that the Gunn rat also excretes substantial amounts of these same products in the dark. This suggests that these derivatives can be formed by catabolic processes as well as by photochemical reactions, presumably by uncharacterized bilirubin oxygenases that are utilized by the Gunn rat for the alternative pathways of bilirubin metabolism.

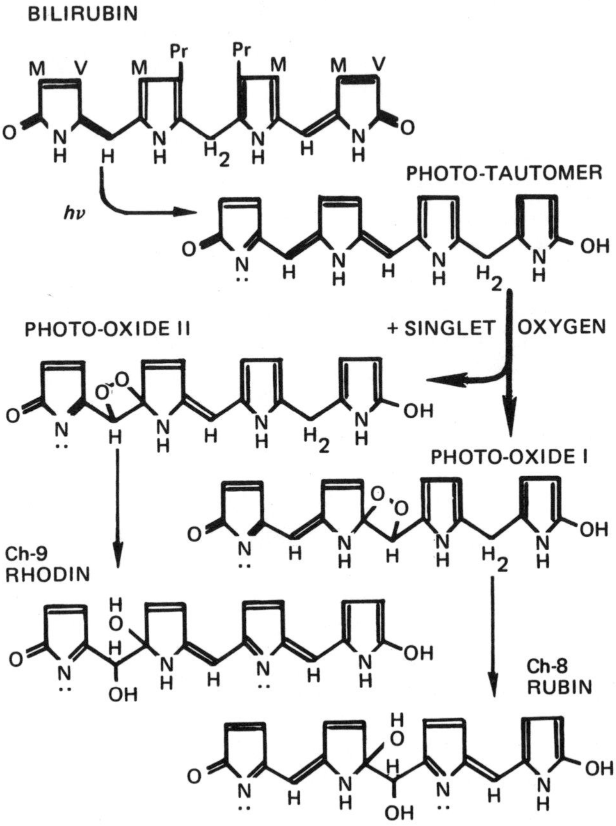

BILIRUBIN

PHOTO-TAUTOMER

PHOTO-OXIDE II

+ SINGLET OXYGEN

PHOTO-OXIDE I

Ch-9 RHODIN

Ch-8 RUBIN

FIGURE 7 Diagram of proposed scheme for the formation of C-5/Ch-8 and C-6/Ch-9 via addition of singlet oxygen to a phototautomer of bilirubin, which yields two dioxetane (photooxide) intermediates. β-Side-chains on all molecules, as for bilirubin. Isomers with the added OH groups on the right half of the molecule are not shown. (From Berry *et al.*[8])

Why Do Large Amounts of Unconjugated Bilirubin Appear in the Bile during Phototherapy?

We first conjectured that the permeability of the liver cell was altered, permitting a variety of lipid-soluble compounds to "leak" into the bile, a therapeutically exciting possibility. To test this postulate, we used Gunn rats with cannulated bile ducts and kept them in the dark for 33 h. Six animals were then exposed to light, and five others, which served as controls, were kept under dim light throughout the remainder of the experiment. Bile was analyzed for diazo-reactive material,[26] bile salts,[2] cholesterol,[1] and phospholipid.[11] As shown in Figure 8, both groups exhibited a decrease in excretion of bile salts with partial recovery to a new plateau by the end of 33 h. This is the characteristic response of the rat to interruption of the enterohepatic circulation.[5] Phototherapy applied during the recovery plateau did not alter the excretion of bile salts, although the usual striking increase in excretion of diazo-reactive material occurred. As shown in Table 1, similar patterns were observed is the excretion of cholesterol and phospholipids, which were likewise unaltered by phototherapy. Phototherapy applied during the nadir of excretion from 11 to 27 h likewise did not alter the output of these micellar components of bile. Apparently, phototherapy did not cause the liver to become abnormally permeable to lipid-soluble substances.

A second possibility, suggested by Dr. Barbara Billing, was that the liver had become permeable to albumin, which was leaking into the bile together with bound bilirubin. Since bilirubin interferes with the measure-

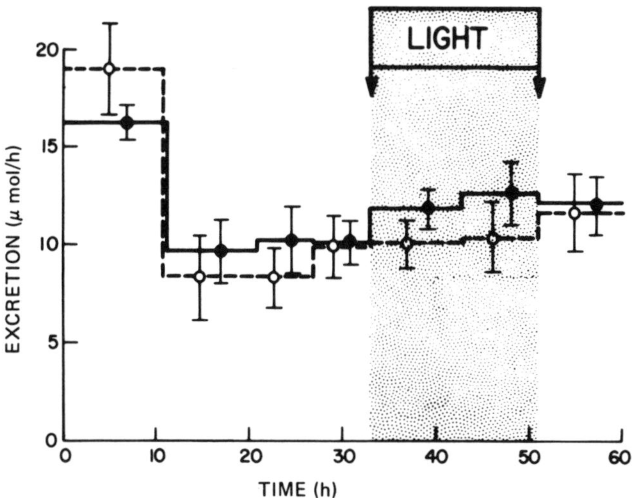

FIGURE 8 Effect of phototherapy on excretion of bile salts in Gunn rat bile. Total bile salt output in micromoles per hour (mean ± SE) shown at different intervals following total biliary diversion at time 0. Five control rats (—○—) were shaded from light throughout the experiment. Six light-treated rats (—●—) were exposed to phototherapy from 33 to 51 h after bile duct cannulation (shaded area).

TABLE 1 Outputs of Micellar Components and Diazo-Reactivity in Gunn Rat Bile (Mean ± SE)

		Hours after Bile-Duct Cannulation						
Component	Phototherapy (h)	0–11	11–21	21–27	27–33	33–43	43–51	51–59
Bile salts	None (control) [a]	19.0 ± 2.3	8.5 ± 2.0	8.4 ± 1.5	10.0 ± 1.6	10.1 ± 1.3	10.4 ± 1.8	11.7 ± 1.9
(μmol/h)	33–51 [a]	16.2 ± 1.9	9.7 ± 1.6	10.2 ± 1.7	10.1 ± 1.1	11.9 ± 1.0	12.7 ± 1.6	12.1 ± 1.5
	11–27 [a]	18.7 ± 2.4	9.9 ± 2.2	11.1 ± 1.9	11.9 ± 2.1	9.6 ± 1.5		
Phospholipids	None (control)	2.59 ± .53	0.50 ± .25	0.39 ± 1.0	0.85 ± .09	1.56 ± .22	1.47 ± .20	1.59 ± .23
(μmol/h)	33–51	2.47 ± .30	0.73 ± .29	0.65 ± .24	1.08 ± .33	1.59 ± .31	1.13 ± .39	1.16 ± .40
	11–27	2.84 ± .61	0.90 ± .32	0.69 ± .26	1.02 ± .32	1.28 ± .31		
Cholesterol	None (control)	0.31 ± .06	0.11 ± .03	0.11 ± .04	0.15 ± .02	0.26 ± .03	0.25 ± .04	0.32 ± .03
(μmol/h)	33–51	0.31 ± .04	0.14 ± .02	0.15 ± .02	0.19 ± .03	0.28 ± .03	0.28 ± .05	0.29 ± .05
	11–27	0.35 ± .07	0.15 ± .04	0.17 ± .04	0.16 ± .04	0.25 ± .04		
Diazo-reaction	None (control)	0.19 ± .01	0.13 ± .02	0.14 ± .02	0.14 ± .01	0.16 ± .02	0.16 ± .03	0.18 ± .01
(OD × ml/h)	33–51	0.21 ± .03	0.15 ± .01	0.16 ± .02	0.19 ± .02	0.65 ± .06 [b]	0.65 ± .09 [b]	0.32 ± .02 [b]
	11–27	0.21 ± .04	0.31 ± .03 [b]	0.55 ± .08 [b]	0.25 ± .03	0.15 ± .03		

[a] Number of animals studied: controls (no phototherapy), 5; phototherapy from 33 to 51 h after bile duct cannulation, 6; phototherapy from 11 to 27 h after bile duct cannulation, 3.

[b] Values significantly different from control animals ($p < 0.02$) by student "t-test" with Yates's correction for small groups.[16]

ment of protein in bile by the biuret [19] or Lowry method,[24] we used the subterfuge of injecting Evans blue intravenously into these animals. This dye binds very tightly, although incompletely, to the plasma albumin [3] but normally appears in the bile in only very small quantities.[27] In both Gunn rats studied, there was an exponential decline in the concentration of Evans blue in the plasma as it gradually diffused into the tissues (Figure 9). Phototherapy produced no break in this plasma-decay curve,

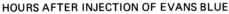

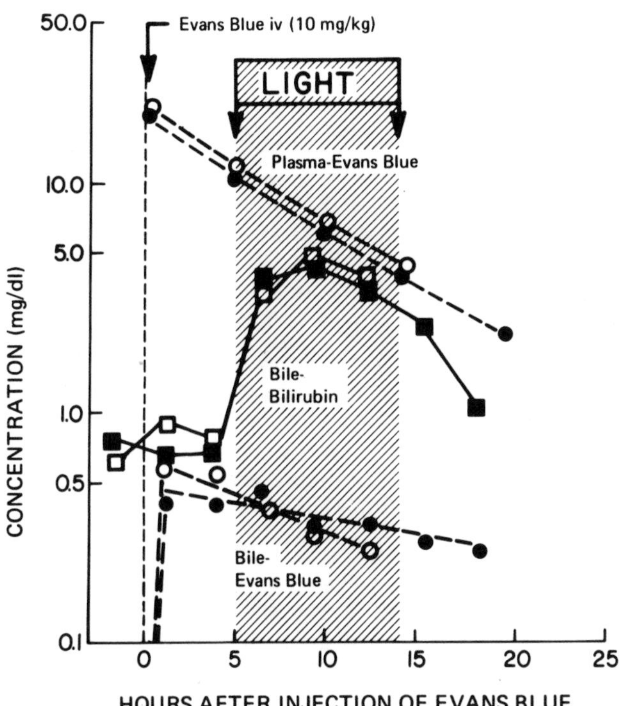

FIGURE 9 Effect of phototherapy on excretion of Evans blue and bilirubin in the bile of two Gunn rats. Rats were provided with an external biliary fistula 3 h prior to intravenous injection of Evans blue, 10 mg/kg, at time 0. Phototherapy was applied from 5 to 14 h later (cross-hatched area). Serial changes in concentrations of Evans blue (—○—●—) in plasma and bile (OD at 615 and 610 nm, respectively) and of bilirubin in bile (—■—□—) (OD at 450 nm of the lower phase from a Folch solvent-partition of bile) are plotted semilogarithmically for each animal. Bile catheter of the rat represented by the open symbols plugged at the fifteenth hour.

nor did it engender an increase in the concentration of Evans blue in the bile at a time when the concentration of bile bilirubin rose precipitously. Gel electrophoresis [14] demonstrated that the Evans blue in the plasma remained bound to albumin during phototherapy. This experiment thus provided no evidence for alteration in hepatic permeability to Evans blue or to the albumin to which it was attached.

We next wondered whether the polar photoproducts might be carrying bilirubin into the bile by complex formation as occurs when conjugated bilirubin is injected into the Gunn rat.[10] Photoproducts were prepared in donor Gunn rats exposed to light and then injected into recipient Gunn rats kept in the dark. The donor rats, previously given ^{3}H-bilirubin, were exposed to phototherapy and the labeled photoproducts were isolated from their bile by the solvent-partition techniques described earlier. The tritiated photoproducts were then administered intravenously to two recipient Gunn rats that had previously received ^{14}C-bilirubin to label their endogenous pigment pool. The recipient rats were kept in the dark and their bile was subjected to radioassay to determine the rate of excretion of ^{3}H-labeled exogenous pigments and ^{14}C-labeled endogenous pigments. Isolated fractions of tritiated bilirubin derivatives, each representing pigments derived from 10 h of bile output by a donor rat, were sequentially injected intravenously at 6-hour intervals. Eight hours after injection of the last of the four pigment fractions, the recipient rats were exposed to light for 14 h to demonstrate their capability for enhanced excretion of bilirubin and radioactivity during phototherapy.

Excretion of the exogenous tritium-labeled derivatives is shown in Figure 10. After injection of either the polar bilirubin derivatives excreted by the Gunn rat in the dark (the D-fractions) or the photoderivatives excreted by the Gunn rat under phototherapy (the L-fractions), over 80 percent of the tritium label was excreted in 2 h and another 10 percent or more appeared within the next 2 h. This is the first direct demonstration that the photoproducts are excreted rapidly in the bile, an important observation since the pigments in the two S-fractions are lipid-soluble at pH 7, making it possible for them to diffuse into the brain had they been retained in the body.

Figure 11 shows the biliary excretion of ^{14}C-labeled endogenous pigments by the two recipient Gunn rats. It is evident that none of the injections of polar bilirubin derivatives, either from light or dark bile fractions, led to any increase in the excretion of endogenous ^{14}C-labeled pigments. Thus, the hepatic transport of photoderivatives did not mediate the excretion of endogenous bilirubin in the bile. By contrast, as shown on the right, phototherapy of the recipient Gunn rats induced a clear-cut increase in the output of ^{14}C radioactivity (and also of diazoreactivity), demonstrating that they were capable of responding to photo-

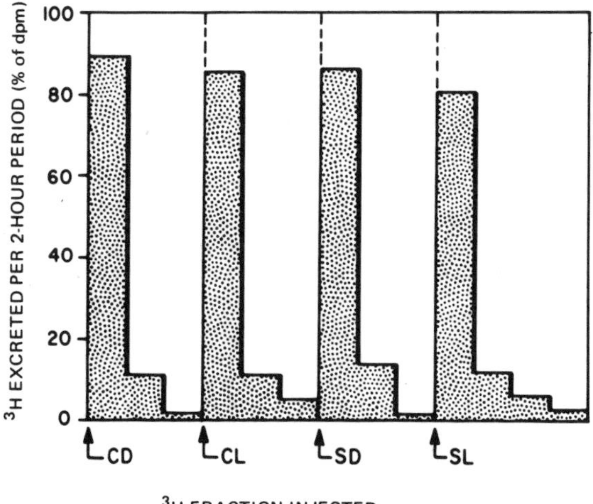

FIGURE 10 Excretion of administered ^{3}H-bilirubin derivatives in the bile of recipient Gunn rats, expressed as the percentage of the total radioactivity excreted during the 6 h after administration of each pigment fraction. Each bar represents a 2-hour period. The labeled pigment fractions were isolated by solvent partition (*see* Figures 2 and 3) of bile collected from donor Gunn rats during a period under dim light (D) or during phototherapy (L). C refers to C-fractions, and S to methanol-soluble material from F-fractions of the respective donor bile samples. The donor rats had been given ^{3}H-bilirubin intravenously before bile collections began.

therapy with the expected augmented excretion of endogenous pigments.

This last experiment permits two conclusions. The first is that the bilirubin derivatives and photoproducts produced by the Gunn rat *in vivo* are rapidly and efficiently excreted in the bile and are therefore presumably without glucuronide conjugation. Such rapid clearance from the body would render toxicity from these products unlikely. The second conclusion is that excretion of these polar photoproducts does not mediate the observed outpouring of unconjugated bilirubin that occurs during phototherapy. The mechanism of this remarkable excretion of unconjugated bilirubin remains a mystery.

Acknowledgments

We thank Mrs. Regina Longyear for her assistance with the chemical assays of bile, and Miss Bernice Branch of the Skin and Cancer Hospital, Temple University Health Sciences Center, for providing the Gunn rats.

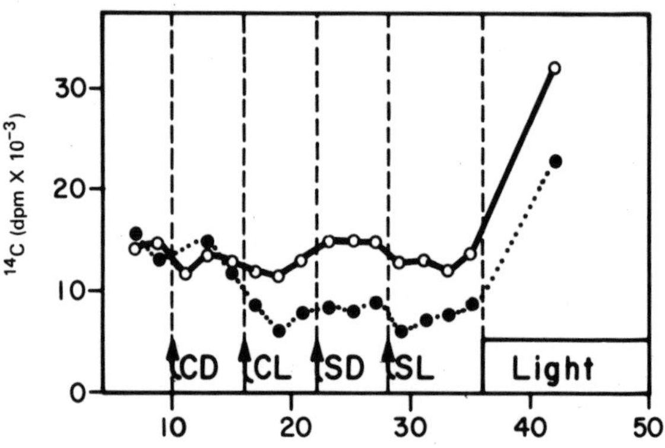

FIGURE 11 Biliary excretion of endogenous ^{14}C bile pigments by recipient Gunn rats following intravenous injection of ^{14}C-bilirubin at time 0, and subsequent injection of exogenous ^{3}H-bilirubin derivatives at 6–hour intervals, as illustrated in Figure 10. Each curve represents the excretion of ^{14}C radioactivity in 2–hour bile collection periods. The rats were maintained under dim light for the first 36 h, then exposed to phototherapy for 14 h.

REFERENCES

1. Abell, L. L., B. B. Levy, B. B. Brodie, and F. E. Kendall. A simplified method for the estimation of total cholesterol in serum and demonstration of its specificity. J. Biol. Chem. 195:357–366, 1952.
2. Admirand, W. H., and D. M. Small. The physicochemical basis of cholesterol gallstone formation in man. J. Clin. Invest. 47:1043–1052, 1968.
3. Allen, T. H. and P. D. Orahovats. Combination of toluidine dye isomers with plasma albumin. Am. J. Physiol. 161:473–482, 1950.
4. Arias, I. M., L. Johnson, and S. Wolfson. Biliary excretion of injected conjugated and unconjugated bilirubin by normal and Gunn rats. Am. J. Physiol. 200:1091–1094, 1961.
5. Balint, J. A., D. A. Beeler, E. C. Kyriakides, and D. H. Treble. The effect of bile salts upon lecithin synthesis. J. Lab. Clin. Med. 77:122–133, 1971.
6. Bernstein, L. H., J. Ben Ezzer, L. Gartner, and I. M. Arias. Hepatic intracellular distribution of tritium-labeled unconjugated and conjugated bilirubin in normal and Gunn rats. J. Clin. Invest. 45:1194–1201, 1966.
7. Bernstein, R. B., M. J. Novy, G. J. Piasecki, R. Lester, and B. T. Jackson. Bilirubin metabolism in the fetus. J. Clin. Invest. 48:1678–1688, 1969.
8. Berry, C. S., J. E. Zarembo, and J. D. Ostrow. Evidence for conversion of bilirubin to dihydroxyl derivatives in the Gunn rat. Biochem. Biophys. Res. Commun. 49:1366–1375, 1972.

9. Broughton, P. M. G., E. J. R. Rossiter, C. B. M. Warren, G. Goulis, and P. S. Lord. Effect of blue light on hyperbilirubinaemia. Arch. Dis. Child. 40:666–671, 1965.
10. Callahan, E. W., Jr., and R. Schmid. Excretion of unconjugated bilirubin in the bile of Gunn rats. Gastroenterology 57:134–137, 1969.
11. Chen, P. S., Jr., T. Y. Toribara, and H. Warner. Microdetermination of phosphorus. Anal. Chem. 28:1756–1758, 1956.
12. Cremer, R. J., D. W. Perryman, and D. H. Richards. Influence of light on the hyperbilirubinaemia of infants. Lancet 1:1094–1097, 1958.
13. Davies, R. E., and S. J. Keohane. Some aspects of the photochemistry of bilirubin. Boll. Chim. Farm. 109:589–598, 1970.
14. Davis, B. J. Disk electrophoresis. II. Method and application to human serum proteins. Ann. N.Y. Acad. Sci. 121:404–427, 1964.
15. Diamond, I., and R. Schmid. Neonatal hyperbilirubinemia and kernicterus. Experimental support for treatment by exposure to visible light. Arch. Neurol. 18:699–702, 1968.
16. Edwards, A. L. Statistical Methods for the Behavioral Sciences, pp. 246–277. New York: Rinehart and Co., Inc., 1954.
17. Garay, E. A. R., E. V. Flock, and C. A. Owen, Jr. Composition of bile pigments in the Gunn rat. Am. J. Physiol. 210:684–688, 1966.
18. Glauser, S. C., S. A. Lombard, E. M. Glauser, and T. R. C. Sisson. Action spectrum for the photodestruction of bilirubin. Proc. Soc. Exp. Biol. Med. 136:518–519, 1971.
19. Gornall, A. G., C. J. Bardawill, and M. M. David. Determination of serum proteins by means of the biuret reaction. J. Biol. Chem. 177:751–766, 1949.
20. Haddock, J. H., and H. L. Nadler. Bilirubin toxicity in human cultivated fibroblasts and its modification by light treatment. Proc. Soc. Exp. Biol. Med. 134:45–48, 1970.
21. Haslewood, G. A. D. Recent developments in our knowledge of bile salts. Physiol. Rev. 35:178–196, 1955.
22. Lathe, G. H., and M. Walker. The synthesis of bilirubin glucuronide in animal and human liver. Biochem. J. 70:705–712, 1958.
23. Levi, A. J., Z. Gatmaitan, and I. M. Arias. Deficiency of hepatic organic anion-binding protein, impaired organic anion uptake by liver and "physiologic" jaundice in newborn monkeys. N. Engl. J. Med. 283:1136–1139, 1970.
24. Lowry, O. H., N. J. Rosebrough, A. L. Farr, and R. J. Randall. Protein measurement with the Folin phenol reagent. J. Biol. Chem. 193:265–275, 1951.
25. McDonagh, A. F. The role of singlet oxygen in bilirubin photo-oxidation. Biochem. Biophys. Res. Commun. 44:1306–1311, 1971.
26. Michaelsson, M. Bilirubin determination in serum and urine. Studies on diazo methods and a new copper-azo pigment method. Scand. J. Clin. Lab. Invest. 13 (Suppl 56):1–80, 1961.
27. Miller, A. T., Jr. Excretion of the blue dye, T–1824, in the bile. Am. J. Physiol. 151:229–233, 1947.
28. Ostrow, J. D. Photocatabolism of labeled bilirubin in the congenitally jaundiced (Gunn) rat. J. Clin. Invest. 50:707–718, 1971.
29. Ostrow, J. D. Photo-oxidative derivatives of [^{14}C] bilirubin and their excretion by the Gunn rat, pp. 117–127. In I. A. D. Bouchier and B. H. Billing, Eds. Bilirubin Metabolism. Oxford: Blackwell Scientific Publications, 1967.

30. Ostrow, J. D., and C. S. Berry. Effect of phototherapy on hepatic excretory function in normal and Gunn rats. Gastroenterology 62: 168, 1972. (A)
31. Ostrow, J. D., and C. S. Berry. Excretion of exogenous and endogenous bile pigments after intravenous administration of bilirubin photoderivatives to Gunn rats. Gastroenterology 64:152, 1973. (A)
32. Ostrow, J. D., L. Hammaker, and R. Schmid. The preparation of crystalline bilirubin-C^{14}. J. Clin. Invest. 40:1442–1452, 1961.
33. Ostrow, J. D., and N. H. Murphy. Isolation and properties of conjugated bilirubin from bile. Biochem. J. 120:311–327, 1970.
34. Ostrow, J. D., D. C. Nicholson, and M. S. Stoll. Derivatives of the alkaline degradation of bilirubin. Gastroenterology 60:186, 1971. (A)
35. Schmid, R., J. Axelrod, L. Hammaker, and R. L. Swarm. Congenital jaundice in rats, due to a defect in glucuronide formation. J. Clin. Invest. 37:1123–1130, 1958.
36. Schmid, R., and L. Hammaker. Metabolism and disposition of C^{14}-bilirubin in congenital and nonhemolytic jaundice. J. Clin. Invest. 42:1720–1734, 1963.
37. Siedel, W., and E. Grams. Über Bildung und Konstitution der Mesobilipurpurine und Mesocholeteline sowie über eine neue Ausfuhrung der Gmelinschen Reaktion. Z. Physiol. Chem. 267:49–78, 1941.
38. Silberberg, D. H., L. Johnson, H. Schutta, and L. Ritter. Effects of photodegradation products of bilirubin on myelinating cerebellum cultures. J. Pediatr. 77:613–618, 1970.
39. Thaler, M. M. Toxic effects of bilirubin and its photodecomposition products. Birth Defects 6:128–130, 1970.

MARILYN L. COWGER

Toxicity and Protein Binding of Biliverdin and Other Bile Pigments

For some time we have been interested in the mechanism of bilirubin toxicity. In an attempt to learn more about bilirubin, we have compared it with several other bile pigments closely related in structure. These comparisons have included toxicity studies using tissue culture cells,[4] purified respiratory enzymes,[4] and mitochondrial systems.[11] In addition, the protein binding of these pigments has been compared with bilirubin binding,[8, 9] using analytical ultracentrifugation, Sephadex gel G-150 thin layer chromatography, optical rotatory dispersion (ORD), and circular dichroism (CD) techniques.

One of the pigments compared with bilirubin was biliverdin. Since biliverdin appears to be one product of the photooxidation of bilirubin, at least in some *in vitro* systems,[5, 10, 14] and since the information derived may have clinical implications, this particular pigment was studied in detail. This paper will present some of these comparative investigations of the bile pigments, emphasizing those concerned with biliverdin. In any discussion concerning the possible toxic effect of a product of bilirubin photooxidation, it is not enough to consider only whether the isolated product is toxic; it must also be determined whether the product binds

---

This research was supported by NIH Research Grant HD–05333. The author is a recipient of Research Career Development Award K04 HD 28113.

to albumin. Furthermore, one must ask whether there are any other characteristics of a given product that can in any way enhance the toxicity of bilirubin. These questions will be considered in this discussion. Certain studies involving bilirubin will be reviewed in order to set the proper background for a comparison of the other pigments.

The structures of the four pigments to be discussed are shown in Figure 1. *l*-Stercobilin differs from bilirubin in having 10 more hydro-

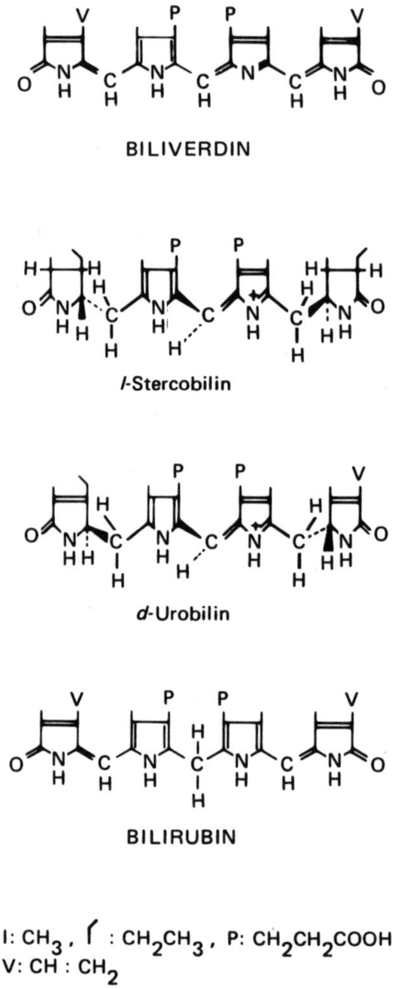

BILIVERDIN

l-Stercobilin

d-Urobilin

BILIRUBIN

I: CH_3, ⌐ : CH_2CH_3, P: CH_2CH_2COOH
V: CH : CH_2

FIGURE 1 Structural formulas for four bile pigments: biliverdin, *l*-stercobilin, *d*-urobilin, and bilirubin.

gens, and the end rings are saturated. *d*-Urobilin has four more hydrogens than bilirubin. Biliverdin has two fewer hydrogens that bilirubin and is formally symmetric. The system is fully conjugated.

Materials and Methods

Bilirubin was a product of Schwarz–Mann. *l*-Stercobilin was obtained by extracting the feces of a patient with congenital erythropoietic porphyria, following the method of Gray and Nicholson.[7] *d*-Urobilin was obtained by a similar method: extracting the feces of a patient with a hemolytic anemia who was on antibiotics. Much attention was paid to the preparation of biliverdin, since the preparations we have used in the past—and, we suspect, those of others—have been very inadequate. There has been significant contamination by other products, and varying amounts have been unknowingly esterified. The one available commercial preparation contains only about 50-percent biliverdin. The method of Gray *et al.*[6] was used in preparing the biliverdin, but, at the suggestion of D. C. Nicholson (personal communication), the initial ferric chloride oxidation of bilirubin was carried out in glacial acetic acid rather than methanol; this was done to prevent esterification. The product was recrystallized from chloroform. Crystals prepared by this method had a very high extinction coefficient (79) and an optical density (OD) ratio (380 nm/650 nm) of 4. For more details of the method, see Lee and Cowger.[8]

The preparation of rat-liver mitochondria and brain mitochondria of several species has been described.[11] Methodology for determining oxygen uptake, respiratory control, oxidative phosphorylation, and swelling may be found in that reference. Absorption spectra were recorded on a Cary Model 14 spectrophotometer. ORD was recorded on a Cary 60 spectropolarimeter, and CD was recorded on the same instrument with CD-attachment 6002. For details, see Lee and Cowger[9] and Blauer and King.[2] Sephadex gel G-150 thin-layer chromatography was carried out in the presence of 0.1 *M* phosphate; a running angle of 15 deg and a plate thickness of 0.4 mm were used. A Beckman Model E ultracentrifuge with a photoelectric scanning system was used to study the sedimentation-velocity behavior of the free-pigments bilirubin and biliverdin, each pigment with albumin, and mixtures of the pigments with albumin. A 6-hole rotor was used in sedimenting the solutions in duplicate or triplicate at 40,000 rpm at room temperature for 2½ h and scanned at the OD maxima. The patterns obtained were superimposed in the figures by matching the menisci and the cell bottoms.

The electron micrographs were taken with a Philips electron microscope (Model EM 300) at an accelerating voltage of 60 kV. Samples for sectioning were prepared as follows: Specimens were fixed at 0–4 deg with 1-percent glutaraldehyde for 30 min, then with 1-percent osmium tetroxide (buffered with 50 m*M* phosphate, pH 7.5) for 90 min; dehydrated with various gradations of ethanol; embedded in Epon 812 resin; and sectioned with a Blum ultramicrotome (Model MT-2). Sections (0.4–0.6 μm thick) were stained with 1-percent lead citrate and 1-percent uranyl acetate, successively.

Effects of Bilirubin on Mitochondrial Reactions

Bilirubin has been found to be extremely toxic to isolated systems of rat-liver mitochondria and brain mitochondria from a variety of sources.[11] Bilirubin blocks oxygen uptake, uncouples oxidative phosphorylation, and abolishes respiratory control. Figure 2 shows the effect of bilirubin on the oxygen uptake of rat-liver mitochondria. At low concentrations (that is, less than 20 μM), bilirubin stimulated respiration, and at higher concentrations (greater than 50 μM), it depressed respiration. In this regard, it is similar to some other uncouplers of oxidative phosphorylation. Heart mitochondria responded similarly, demonstrating this biphasic response.

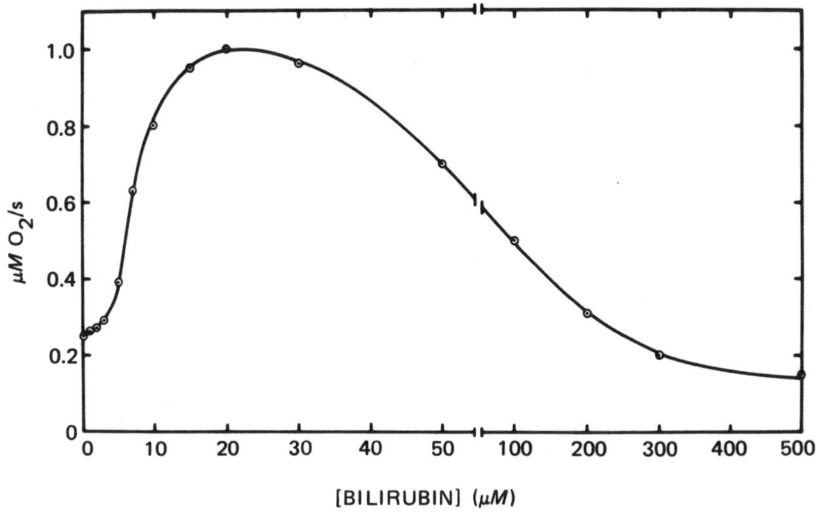

FIGURE 2 Effect of bilirubin on respiration of mitochondria. The system contained 100-m*M* sucrose, 50-m*M* mannitol, 8-m*M* magnesium chloride, 5-m*M* potassium phosphate, 5-m*M* trischloride, 10-m*M* β-hydroxybutyrate, and 0.8-mg rat-liver mitochondrial protein; pH 7.5. (From Mustafa *et al.*[11] Reprinted by permission.)

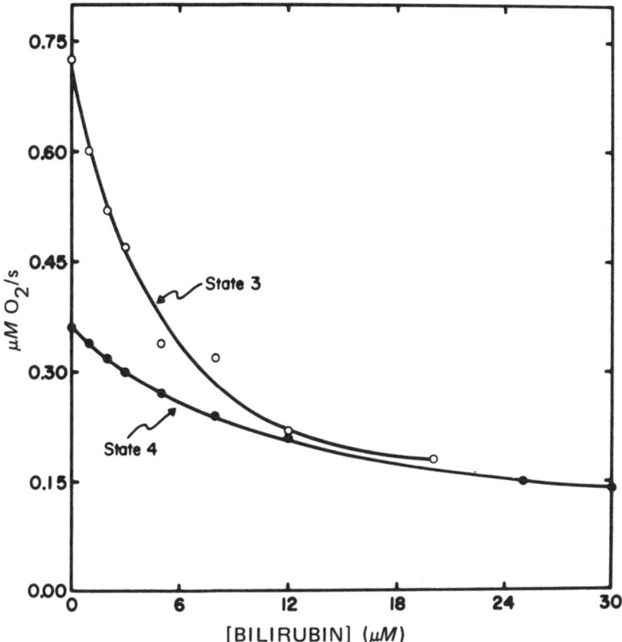

FIGURE 3 Effect of bilirubin on respiration of brain mitochondria. The system contained 3.0-m*M* mannitol, 10-m*M* potassium chloride, 5-m*M* potassium phosphate, 10-m*M* tris-chloride, and 1.5-mg rabbit-brain mitochondrial protein per milliliter; pH 7.5. Other additions were 10-m*M* succinate, 10-m*M* α-glycerophosphate, 100-μM ADP, and bilirubin as indicated. (From Mustafa *et al.*[11] Reprinted by permission.)

In brain it was not possible to demonstrate the biphasic effect. There was no stimulation of respiration, but only inhibition could be demonstrated for succinate or α-glycerophosphate in either State 3 or State 4 (Figure 3). The concentration of bilirubin for 50 percent of the maximal effect (K_m)* was found to be less than 3 μM for State 3 respiration and 5 μM for State 4 respiration for rabbit-brain mitochondria.

Figure 4 depicts the effects of bilirubin on the respiratory control index (RCI) and on phosphorylation as measured by the adenosine diphosphate:oxygen (ADP:O) ratio. Respiratory control was more sensitive to the toxic effect of bilirubin than was phosphorylation. The K_m for the

* K_m in this paper refers to 50 percent of the maximal value as defined in the original work of Mustafa *et al.*[11]

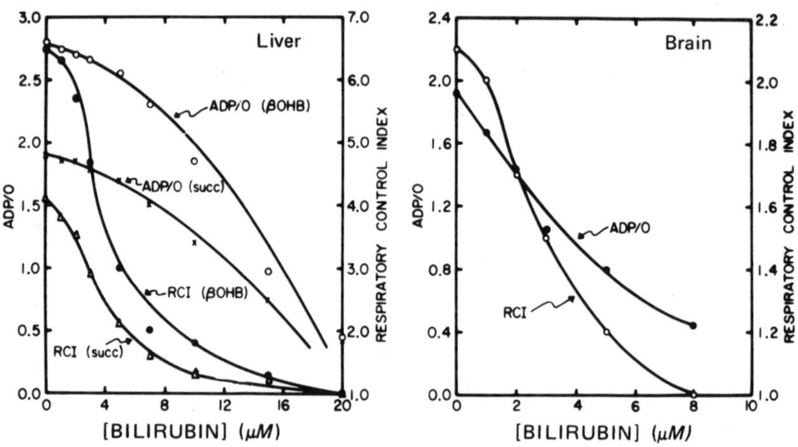

FIGURE 4 Effect of bilirubin on phosphorylation. *Left:* Rat-liver mitochondria. The basal medium contained 180-m*M* sucrose, 18-m*M* mannitol, 8-m*M* magnesium chloride, 5-m*M* potassium phosphate, 5-m*M* trischloride, and 3.6-mg mitochondrial protein per milliliter. Other additions, where made, were 10-m*M* β-hydroxybutyrate (βOHB), 10-m*M* succinate (succ), 150-μ*M* ADP, and bilirubin as indicated. *Right:* Rabbit-brain mitochondria. The conditions were the same as those described in Figure 3. Respiratory control index, RCI. (From Mustafa *et al.*[11] Reprinted by permission.)

RCI for rat-liver mitochondria, with succinate or β-hydroxybutyrate as the substrate was 4-μ*M* bilirubin. In rabbit-brain mitochondria, the K_m for the RCI was 2.5 μ*M* for the substrate combination of succinate and α-glycerophosphate. In the case of phosphorylation, the brain was more sensitive than the liver; at 8-μ*M* bilirubin obliteration of phosphorylation was almost complete in the brain but was less than 50-percent complete in the liver.

In addition to these activities, bilirubin also induced a large-amplitude irreversible swelling of mitochondria. The swelling required an energy source, monovalent cations, and a permeant anion (Figure 5). Swelling was measured as a drop in the OD of the solution at 590 nm. The rate and extent of swelling in liver mitochondria were always higher than those observed in heart and brain mitochondria. For example, 10-μ*M* bilirubin caused an OD change of about 0.8 in liver mitochondria; whereas, under similar conditions, the changes were only about 0.4 and 0.3 for heart and brain, respectively. The K_m for swelling in rat liver was about 2.5-μ*M* bilirubin and, for brain, 2 μ*M*. Electron transport through any segment of the respiratory chain could provide energy

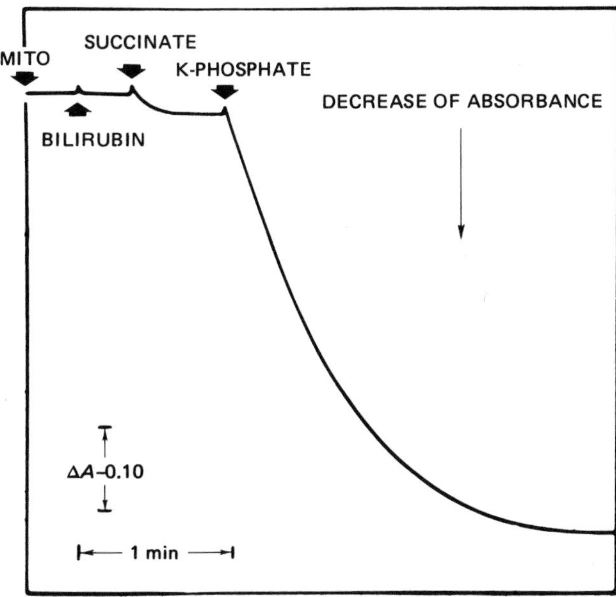

FIGURE 5 Large-amplitude irreversible swelling of rat-liver mitochondria induced by bilirubin. Swelling was measured by recording the decrease in absorbance at 590 nm with a high-intensity light source. The basal medium contained 50-m*M* mannitol, 50-m*M* trischloride (pH 7.5), 7-m*M* magnesium chloride, and about 1-mg rat-liver mitochondrial protein per milliliter. Other additions were 10-μM bilirubin, 10-μM potassium phosphate, and 10-m*M* succinate.

for swelling. Swelling could be inhibited by addition of an uncoupler or a respiratory inhibitor.

Figure 6 shows the morphological change concomitant with this decrease in OD. Figure 6(a) depicts normal beef-heart mitochondria, and Figure 6(b) the same mitochondria following the addition of 10-μM bilirubin. The dense cristae just melted away; some mitochondria lost the outer membrane, and in others the inner membrane also fragmented.

These studies demonstrate what an extremely effective poison bilirubin is. All these effects of bilirubin on mitochondria are membrane-related. Bilirubin has many of the properties of the mitochondrial transport-inducing agents, such as gramicidin, valinomycin, and the nonaction homologues, which increase the permeability of the mitochondrial membrane to alkali cations.[15] However, unlike these agents, bilirubin induces a unidirectional movement of ions and water that leads to an irreversible

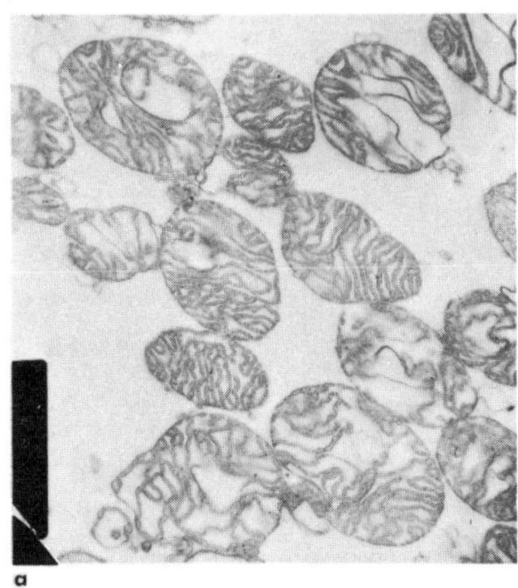

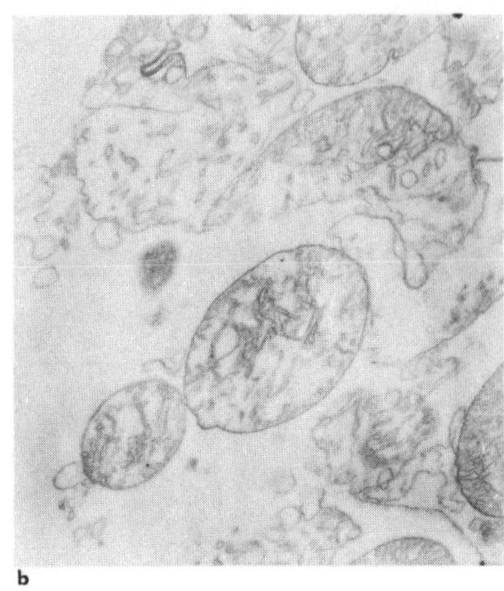

FIGURE 6 (a) Electron micrograph of normal beef-heart mitochondria. Final magnification × 42,000. (b) Electron micrograph of beef-heart mitochondria following the addition of 10-μM bilirubin. Final magnification × 42,000. (From Cowger.[3])

swelling because of the osmotic effect.[11] The addition of bovine serum albumin (BSA) can prevent all these toxic effects of bilirubin.

Mitochondrial Reactions of Biliverdin

Table 1 shows the effects of biliverdin on rat-liver mitochondria. There was no effect on phosphorylation for either succinate or β-hydroxybutyrate oxidation, even up to 400-μM biliverdin in the case of succinate. With succinate as a substrate, there was about a 40-percent decrease of RCI at 400-μM biliverdin; thus, if one wished to produce, with this biliverdin preparation, an effect comparable with the effect of a given amount of bilirubin on RCI, the amount of the biliverdin preparation would have to be more than 100 times as great as the amount of bilirubin.

The biliverdin preparation did appear to exert some effect on State 3 oxidation of succinate, which began dropping at a concentration of about 150-μM biliverdin. State 3 was inhibited about 35 percent by 400-μM biliverdin. With β-hydroxybutyrate there was only a questionable effect on State 3 oxidation at 200-μM biliverdin.

The inhibitory effects seen with these very high concentrations of pigment pose some problems in interpretation. We cannot ascribe all these effects to biliverdin without serious reservations. It appears impossible to

TABLE 1 Effect of Biliverdin on Rat-Liver Mitochondria [a]

Mitochondria	Addition	O_2 Uptake (μM/min) no ADP	O_2 Uptake (μM/min) + ADP	ADP:O Ratio	Respiratory Control Index
Rat liver (1.1 mg protein per ml)	1. Succinate [b]	23	126	1.8	5.5
	2. 1+Biliverdin, 20 μM	22	122	1.6	5.5
	3. 1+Biliverdin, 40 μM	23	133	1.6	5.8
	4. 1+Biliverdin, 80 μM	22	120	1.7	5.7
	5. 1+Biliverdin, 100 μM	21	126	1.6	6.0
	6. 1+Biliverdin, 150 μM	21	115	1.8	5.5
	7. 1+Biliverdin, 200 μM	23	106	1.7	4.6
	8. 1+Biliverdin, 400 μM	26	83	1.8	3.2
	9. β-Hydroxybutyrate [c]	11	38	2.3	3.4
	10. 9+Biliverdin, 20 μM	9	41	2.6	4.6
	11. 9+Biliverdin, 40 μM	10	34	2.7	3.4
	12. 9+Biliverdin, 60 μM	10	36	2.8	3.4
	13. 9+Biliverdin, 100 μM	10	36	2.6	3.6
	14. 9+Biliverdin, 200 μM	10	31	2.8	3.0

[a] The basal medium included 230-mM mannitol, 70-mM sucrose, 20-mM tris-HCl, 20-mM EDTA, 5-mM potassium phosphate, and mitochondria, pH 7.4. Other additions were 10-mM succinate and 10-mM β-hydroxybutyrate.

[b] Average of four determinations.

[c] Average of two determinations.

obtain absolutely pure biliverdin. At high concentrations of the pigment, contaminants present in small amounts may become significant, or there may be other nonspecific effects. Suppose there is a bilirubin contamination of about 1 percent, a very likely possibility. Since K_m for the RCI for bilirubin with these substrates is about 4 μM, such contamination might explain the 40-percent drop seen at about 400-μM biliverdin. The decrease in the ADP:O ratio at 4-μM bilirubin is only about 10 percent. Perhaps we did not detect this small change in this particular experiment. The results of the experiment suggest that bilirubin contamination could not have been higher than about 1 percent; if it had been higher, we would have seen more serious effects on the mitochondria even at much lower concentrations of biliverdin.

Table 2 shows similar data for rat-brain mitochondria. A substrate system of pyruvate-malate was used to evaluate the NADH pathway; RCI at 400-μM biliverdin was decreased by about 45 percent. The ADP:O ratio in the case of brain was decreased by about 30 percent, and the State 3 respiration was depressed about 38 percent. The drop in the

TABLE 2 Effect of Biliverdin on Rat-Brain Mitochondria [a]

Mitochondria	Addition	O_2 Uptake (μM/min) no ADP	O_2 Uptake (μM/min) + ADP	ADP:O Ratio	Respiratory Control Index
Rat brain (0.98 mg protein per ml)	1. Pyruvate-malate [b]	4.0	18.7	2.1	4.7
	2. 1+Biliverdin, 25 μM	4.2	17.5	2.0	4.2
	3. 1+Biliverdin, 50 μM	3.2	17.0	2.0	5.2
	4. 1+Biliverdin, 75 μM	3.2	17.0	2.0	5.2
	5. 1+Biliverdin, 100 μM	3.8	16.0	2.0	4.3
	6. 1+Biliverdin, 150 μM	3.0	14.5	1.9	4.8
	7. 1+Biliverdin, 200 μM	2.6	13.0	2.2	5.0
	8. 1+Biliverdin, 300 μM	6.5	15.0	1.8	2.3
	9. 1+Biliverdin, 400 μM	5.0	12.5	1.5	2.5
Rat brain (0.60 mg protein per ml)	10. Succinate [c]	10.2	27.7	1.4	2.8
	11. 10+Biliverdin, 20 μM	10.1	28.6	1.4	2.9
	12. 10+Biliverdin, 50 μM	11.0	19.8	1.6	1.8
	13. 10+Biliverdin, 75 μM	5.5	13.5	1.3	2.5
	14. 10+Biliverdin, 100 μM	13.0	13.0	0	—

[a] The basic conditions were as in Table 1. Other additions included 10-mM succinate and 10-mM pyruvate together with 2-mM malate.

[b] Average of two runs.

[c] Average of five runs.

ADP:O ratio appeared to have begun at about 300-μM biliverdin. With succinate as a substrate, the results were a little different. At 50-μM biliverdin, State 3 oxidation was inhibited 28 percent and RCI was decreased about 36 percent; but, when 100-μM biliverdin was reached, respiratory control and phosphorylation were obliterated.

If contamination of the biliverdin with bilirubin was only about 1 percent or less, we cannot explain this effect on the oxidation of succinate by the brain as due wholly to bilirubin contamination. If we ascribe the whole effect to biliverdin, it still takes about 12 times more biliverdin than bilirubin to achieve a similar effect in brain. At any rate, we feel reasonably safe in saying that biliverdin is a far less effective biological poison than bilirubin if it has any significant toxicity at all.

Biliverdin did not induce swelling of rat-liver mitochondria, even at concentrations up to 240 μM. Indeed, biliverdin appeared to inhibit swelling by bilirubin, although it took a fairly high concentration to do so. At 240-μM biliverdin, swelling due to bilirubin (20 μM) was decreased by about 23 percent. *l*-Stercobilin also did not induce swelling, and 145-μM stercobilin decreased bilirubin swelling by about 50 percent.

Reactions of Bilirubin with Lipid

Another comparison that may shed some light on the difference in toxicity of the bile pigments bilirubin, biliverdin, and stercobilin is the ability to complex with a lipid.[12] Bilirubin appeared to form some kind of complex with a lipid as judged spectrophotometrically (Figure 7). Bilirubin underwent a red-shift in the absorption maximum from 440 to 453, with a pronounced shoulder at 490. Curve A is ordinary alkaline bili-

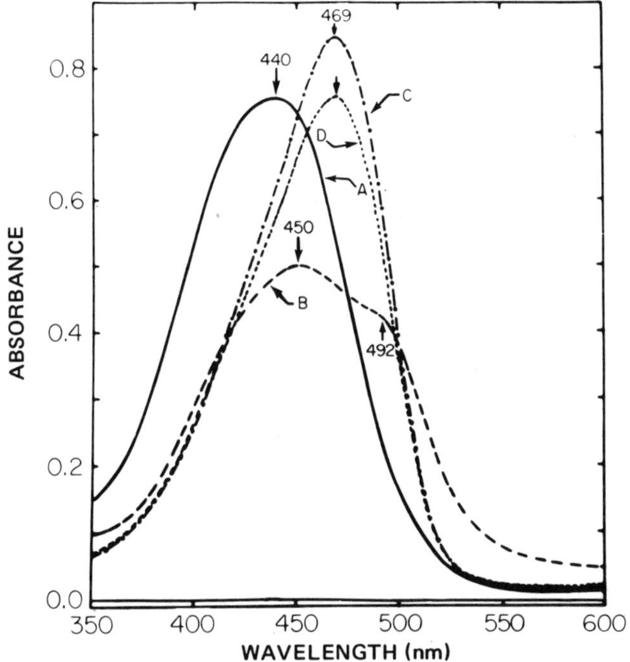

FIGURE 7 Effect of mitochondrial lipid on the absorption spectrum of bilirubin. Curve A contained 50-m*M* potassium phosphate, 50-m*M* trischloride (pH 7.5), and 13.2-μM bilirubin; Curve B contained, in addition, 15-μg mitochondrial lipid. Curve C contained 13.2-μM bilirubin and 6-mg bovine serum albumin per milliliter. Curve D is the same as Curve B but also with 6-mg bovine serum albumin per milliliter. Curve B is qualitatively the same regardless of the source of lipid (mitochondrial lipid, ascites-cell lipid, asolectin, triolein, vegetable oil, lecithin, or linoleic ethyl ester) or lipoidal material (mitochondria, ascites-cell membrane, red-cell membranes, or tissue-culture-cell membranes).

rubin, and Curve B is bilirubin following the addition of lipid—in this case mitochondrial lipid. Curve C is bilirubin plus BSA. Curve D is the addition of albumin to the bilirubin–lipid complex, with the reappearance of the typical bilirubin–albumin complex. Biliverdin and stercobilin did not form a lipid complex, as judged spectrophotometrically at pH 7.5.

The effect of bilirubin with lipid seemed relatively nonspecific. Any number of lipids showed this spectrophotometric change with bilirubin, including mitochondrial lipid, the lipid of ascites cells, asolectin, triolein, vegetable oil, linoleic ethyl ester, and lecithin. The same complex was formed with lipoidal tissues, such as mitochondrial suspensions, red-cell membranes, ascites-cell membranes, and tissue-culture cells. Evidence suggested that bilirubin was bound to mitochondrial lipid rather than mitochondrial protein.[12] Mitochondria extracted free of their lipid did not form this complex. Lipid added to mitochondria partly alleviated the toxic effects of bilirubin on mitochondria. It is speculated that the binding of mitochondrial lipid by bilirubin alters the membrane, leading to a loss of selective permeability to ions so that swelling results. Low concentrations of bilirubin stimulated respiration, giving rise to uncoupled mitochondria, an ion-transport-dependent uncoupling like that of the other transport-inducing agents. With high bilirubin concentration, the lipid essential to the respiratory enzymes was also bound so that respiration was inhibited. The other bile pigments, biliverdin and *l*-stercobilin, are much more water-soluble (as will be discussed later) and appeared neither to form this lipid complex nor to exert much in the way of toxic effects on mitochondria.

Protein Binding of Bilirubin

There is, of course, no question about the binding of bilirubin to serum albumin, and many studies are addressed to this particular point.[13, 16] One such study of the bilirubin–albumin complex was carried out by Blauer and King,[2] who used ORD techniques. Bilirubin by itself is optically inactive. However, the complex of bilirubin and BSA at pH 5 exhibited probably the largest Cotton effect ever recorded, with a peak at 435 nm and a trough at 485–487 nm (Curve A in Figure 8). At pH 7.5 (Curve B), the effect was much diminished. Thus, on binding to BSA, a dissymmetric conformation of the bilirubin molecule was formed, and this conformation was modified by pH. The addition of salt did not affect the Cotton effect at pH 5, but the Cotton effect at pH 7.5 was greatly reduced by 0.1 *M* sodium chloride. Blauer *et al.* recently published a report on a similar study, in which human serum albumin was used.[1]

Protein Binding of Biliverdin, l-*Stercobilin, and* d-*Urobilin*

In the case of the other bile pigments, very little has been written concerning the possibility of their binding to proteins. Consequently, it was necessary to determine whether binding actually occurred. Unlike bilirubin, *l*-stercobilin and *d*-urobilin are optically active. By absorption spectrophotometry, the addition of BSA to stercobilin caused a shift of

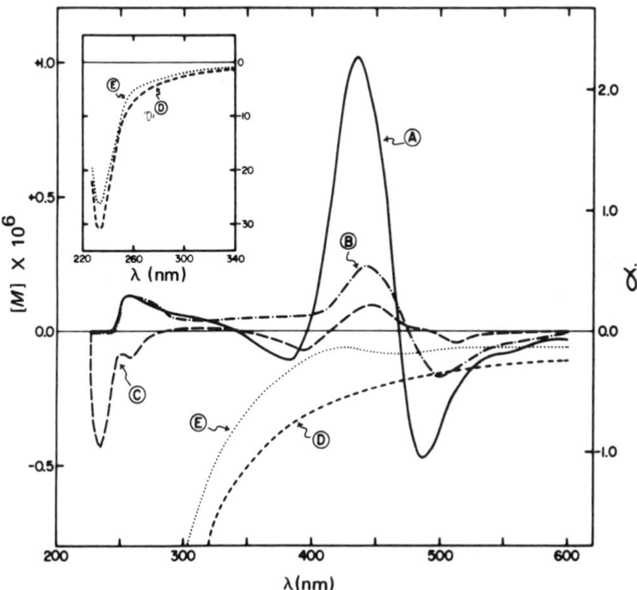

FIGURE 8 ORD of bilirubin in the presence of BSA at different pH values. Left ordinate, molar rotation [*M*] based on total bilirubin for Curves A, B, and C only. Right ordinate, α in degrees per dm for all curves including inset. Protein rotations obtained at the same concentration, pH, and temperature were deducted from total rotation observed for Curves A, B, and C in both presentations. Bilirubin, 22–23 μ*M*; BSA, 3.6 mg/ml (51 μ*M*); temperature, 24.5 ± 1.5 °C. Curve A (bilirubin + BSA), pH 5.0 ± 0.5; Curve B (bilirubin + BSA), pH 7.5 ± 0.1; Curve C (bilirubin + BSA), pH 3.5 ± 0.1; Curve D (BSA), pH 5.0 or 7.5; Curve E (BSA), pH 3.5. *See also* the insets for D and E. Measurements in 0.1-cm cells were completed within about 90 min after mixing the components. Final solutions contained varying amounts (about 1 m*M*) of Cl^- and Na^+ ions. (From Blauer and King.[2] Reprinted by permission.)

less than 1 nm across the pH scale. However, the addition of BSA to *l*-stercobilin and *d*-urobilin by CD techniques (Figure 9) induced a large, negative Cotton effect in the 490-nm region, maximal around pH 4.5, and tapering off sharply on either side of that pH.[9] Figure 9 shows the CD spectra of 19-μM *l*-stercobilin (Curve L-b) in the presence of 410-μM BSA; Curve D-b depicts *d*-urobilin in BSA at about the same concentrations. At pH 4.5, 0.1 *M* sodium chloride abolished the initial interaction of these pigments with protein; at pH 7.5, salt partly recovered the reaction. Thus, the initial binding of these particular pigments may be ionic. For a further discussion of these curves, see Lee and Cowger.[9]

Biliverdin is an optically symmetric molecule, and the changes in absorption characteristics of biliverdin upon the addition of protein were very small. Figure 10 shows the CD spectra of biliverdin and the variation of the Cotton effect with pH.[8] The solid line depicts 14-μM biliverdin at pH 4.5; the BSA : pigment ratio is 0.5. BSA induced large Cotton effects in this symmetric molecule, negative at 650 nm and positive at 380 nm. Once again, maximal induction was seen at pH 4.5; the initial interaction with biliverdin appeared to be two molecules of the pigment to one of the protein, at least at low protein concentrations. Salt drastically diminished the positive Cotton effect in the region of pH 4.5. Lee and Cowger [8] discuss these curves in detail.

Thus, it is fairly clear that all the pigments bind to serum albumin. The protein is dictating the conformation of the pigment. However, it did

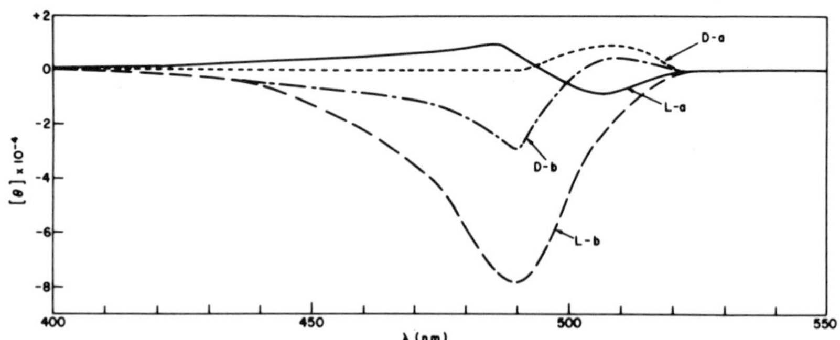

FIGURE 9 Effect of BSA on CD spectra of *l*-stercobilin and *d*-urobilin, pH 4.5. (L-a) free *l*-stercobilin, 19 μM; (L-b) the same in the presence of 410–μM BSA; (D-a) free *d*-urobilin, 15 μM; (D-b) the same in the presence of 440–μM BSA. [Reproduced with permission from PJD Publications Ltd., Westbury, N.Y.; from *Research Communications in Chemical Pathology and Pharmacology,* Vol. 4, p. 124 (1972).]

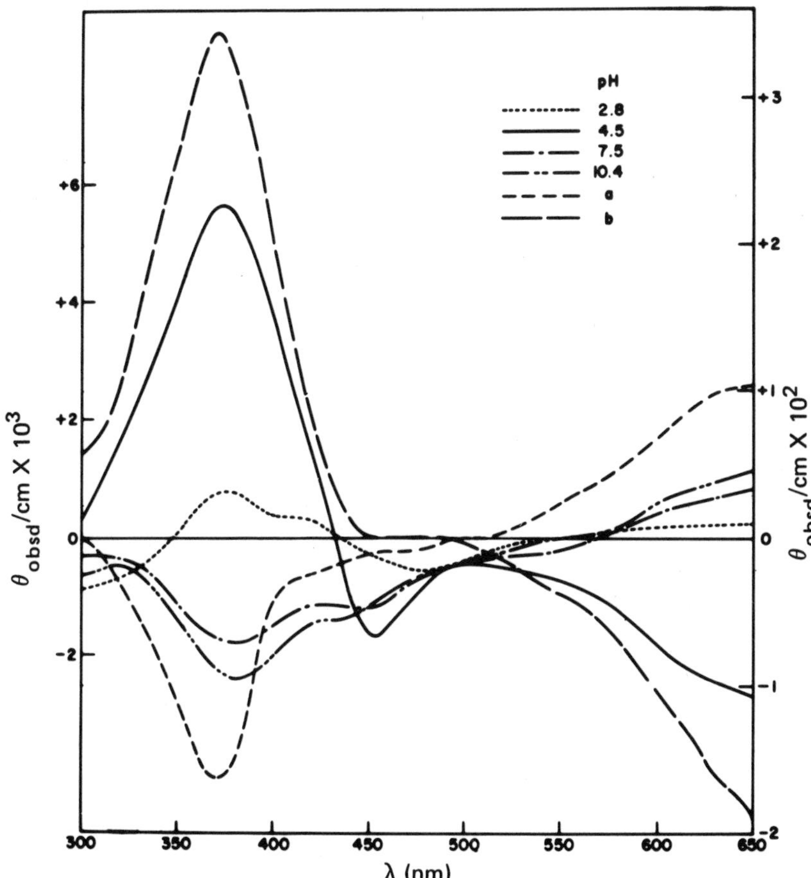

FIGURE 10 CD spectra of biliverdin in the presence of BSA, pH 2.8–10.4, 14-μM biliverdin, range of [BSA]:[Pigment] = 0.48–1.0, average spectra. (a) 75-μM biliverdin solution obtained by magnetically stirring the solid with 320-μM BSA for 1 h and centrifuging the excess solid, pH 4.5, no added electrolyte; (b) 80-μM biliverdin solution in the presence of 32-μM BSA, pH 4.5, [BSA]:[Pigment] = 0.40, [NaCl] ~ 7 mM. [Reproduced with permission from PJD Publications Ltd., Westbury, N.Y.; from *Research Communications in Chemical Pathology and Pharmacology,* Vol. 5, p. 511 (1973).]

not appear that the ORD–CD studies were reflecting the binding in the physiological pH range; other methods were then used to study protein binding at physiological pH 7.4 and to look at the question of what happens to bilirubin binding when the pigments are mixed and the protein is made quite limiting.

Protein Binding of Bile Pigments in Mixed-Pigment Systems

RAT-LIVER MITOCHONDRIA

Various concentrations of biliverdin were preincubated in the dark under nitrogen with 50-μM BSA. Then the mitochondrial reactions with 50-μM bilirubin alone and in combination with 50-μM BSA were observed (Table 3, lines 2 and 3); succinate was used as substrate. The BSA thus was present in an amount calculated theoretically to bind all the bilirubin present in a 1:1 ratio. Upon the addition of bilirubin, phosphorylation and the respiratory control were abolished, as expected, but the addition of BSA restored these functions. Biliverdin (250 μM) depressed State 3 oxidation by 36 percent and RCI by 25 percent; however, phosphorylation was intact. Once again, when albumin was added, the functions were fairly normal (Table 3, lines 4 and 5). Beginning with a 25-μM concentration, biliverdin was added in various amounts in combination with 50-μM BSA, followed by the addition of 50-μM bilirubin, but not until the biliverdin reached 150 μM (or 3 times the bilirubin concentration) was any effect evident on the mitochondria. At 250-μM biliverdin (now 5 times the bilirubin concentration and 5 times the albumin concentration), there appeared to be a decrease of about 40 percent in State 3 oxidation and a decrease of about 25 percent in RCI, but again there was no change in phosphorylation. If these effects are due to some displacement of bilirubin from BSA, it must have been less than 4 or 5 μM, since

TABLE 3 Effect of Mixed-Pigment Systems on Rat-Liver Mitochondria [a]

Mitochondria	Addition	O_2 Uptake (μM/min) no ADP	O_2 Uptake (μM/min) + ADP	ADP:O Ratio	Respiratory Control Index
Rat liver (1.0 mg protein per ml)	1. Succinate	6	47	1.7	7.7
	2. 1+Bilirubin, 50 μM	27	27	—	—
	3. 2+BSA, 50 μM	5	47	1.8	9.1
	4. 1+Biliverdin, 250 μM	5	30	1.8	5.7
	5. 4+Albumin, 50 μM	5	42	2.0	7.7
	6. 3+Biliverdin, 25 μM	5	45	1.8	9.0
	7. 3+Biliverdin, 50 μM	5	42	2.0	8.9
	8. 3+Biliverdin, 100 μM	5	40	1.9	8.2
	9. 3+Biliverdin, 150 μM	4	36	1.9	9.5
	10. 3+Biliverdin, 250 μM	4	25	1.9	6.2
	11. Succinate	5	40	1.9	8.2

[a] The basal conditions were the same as described in Table 1. Other additions were succinate, 10 μM.

we would have found some effect on phosphorylation at that concentration of bilirubin. This experiment suggests that biliverdin in reasonable concentrations does not appear to be influencing the binding of bilirubin to any significant degree. It is certainly not clear from this experiment what is happening to the biliverdin binding. At this particular pH (7.4), there is a significant free solubility of biliverdin; furthermore, as mentioned earlier, there are problems with interpretation at high concentrations of pigment.

SEPHADEX GEL G-150 THIN-LAYER CHROMATOGRAPHY

Another kind of experiment was used to see how biliverdin might be affecting bilirubin binding. Figure 11 shows the results of Sephadex gel

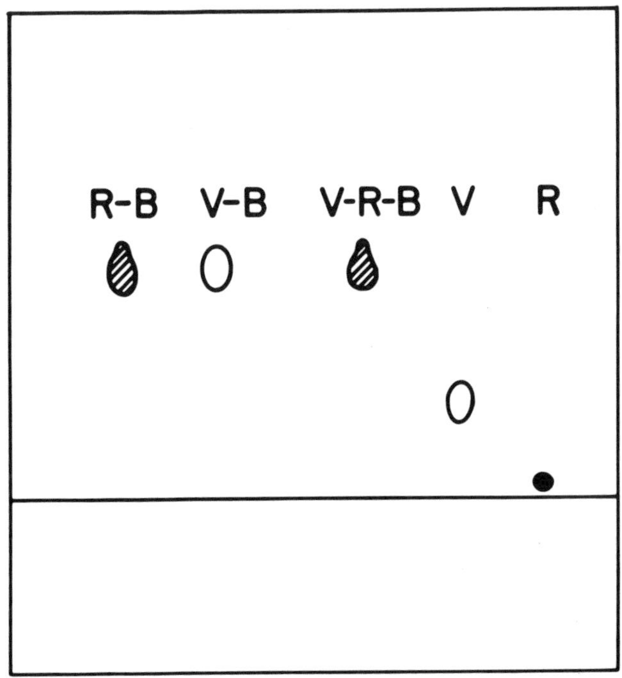

FIGURE 11 Sephadex gel G-150 thin-layer chromatography of bilirubin and biliverdin. A running angle of 15 deg and a plate thickness of 0.4 mm were used in the presence of 0.1 *M* sodium phosphate, pH 7.4. (R) 250-μM bilirubin; (V) 250-μM biliverdin; (R-B) 250-μM bilirubin with 250-μM BSA; (V-B) 250-μM biliverdin with 250-μM BSA; (V-R-B) 250-μM bilirubin with 250-μM biliverdin and 250-μM BSA.

G-150 thin-layer chromatography of each pigment (bilirubin and biliverdin), each pigment with protein, and then a mixture of the two pigments with the same amount of protein. After 1½ h, 250-μM bilirubin (or R in the figure) remained about at the origin, whereas, with protein, 250-μM bilirubin migrated with the protein (250-μM BSA-RB). Free biliverdin (V) migrated a short distance from the origin, but in the presence of an equimolar amount of BSA (250 μM), it migrated with the protein (V-B). When the two pigments were together with BSA, in a 1:1:1 mixture, both pigments migrated with the protein. In this plate, and in other plates that were run, the bluish spot in the position of free biliverdin was either much decreased or not visible. It is possible that, because the color of biliverdin is rather weak, some free biliverdin did not migrate in the mixed-pigment system with the protein. It is obvious that some of it in the mixture migrated with the protein. In addition, difference spectra of the two pigments combined plus the protein showed biliverdin unequivocally present in the mixed spot. There did not appear to be any bilirubin left at the origin in the mixed system. Thus, in this system, biliverdin did not appear to be interfering with bilirubin binding, and both pigments appeared to be migrating with the protein.

ANALYTICAL ULTRACENTRIFUGATION

The sedimentation–velocity behavior of the free pigments, bilirubin and biliverdin—each pigment with albumin, and mixtures of the two pigments with albumin—was studied. In the mixed system, biliverdin was added first and then bilirubin. In order to simplify the presentation, the patterns have been superimposed; the sedimentation is from left to right. The systems were scanned at the OD maxima (375 and 650 nm, biliverdin; 460 nm, bilirubin; and 280 nm, protein).

In Figure 12 the open circles depict 14-μM biliverdin (without protein). There was considerable free solubility of the pigment, probably the total biliverdin added. When 14-μM biliverdin was combined with 7-μM BSA (solid line), about half of the pigment migrated with the protein (1:1). At 280 nm (closed circles) the OD level at the meniscus reflected some free biliverdin because of biliverdin's high ultraviolet absorption. The position of the moving boundary at 375 nm closely matched that observed at 280 nm, showing transport of the pigment by the protein. To increase the accuracy for observing at 650 nm, the concentrations in the biliverdin–protein system were doubled. Again, a sedimentation pattern similar to Figure 12(b) appeared (open squares).

Bilirubin at pH 7.5 showed a small free solubility (Figure 13, open circles), although there was indication of a boundary implying aggregation of the bilirubin. At pH 4.5, there was no free solubility of bilirubin

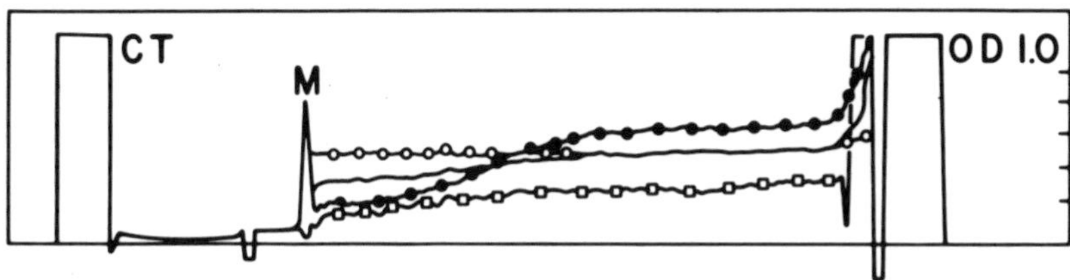

FIGURE 12 Sedimentation–velocity patterns of biliverdin–BSA. CT = cell top, M = meniscus, OD = optical density, the negative deflection = solvent meniscus, 18 °C, pH 7.4, 0.2 *M* phosphate. (a) ○——○, 375 nm, 14-μM biliverdin, no BSA; (b) ————, 375 nm, [Biliverdin]:[BSA] = 14:7 μM; (c) ●——●, 280 nm, Same as b; (d) □——□, 650 nm, [Biliverdin]:[BSA] = 28:14 μM. [Reproduced with permission from PJD Publications Ltd., Westbury, N.Y.; from *Research Communications in Chemical Pathology and Pharmacology*, Vol. 6, p. 624 (1973).]

(data not shown). With the addition of 7-μM BSA at 460 nm (dashed line), the OD level corresponding to the protein boundary showed a tremendous increase. The 280-nanometer pattern was identical to the 460-nanometer pattern.

Figure 14 shows a mixture of the two pigments and protein: 14-μM bilirubin, 14-μM biliverdin, and 7-μM BSA. The meniscus at 375 nm of the mixture, that scanned for biliverdin (solid line), was identical to that of the biliverdin–BSA system alone [Figure 12(b)]. The pattern of the 650-nanometer scan was also identical, although this OD level was smaller than the one in Figure 12(d), which represents 14-μM biliverdin. It thus appears that biliverdin binding in the mixture is unaffected by the presence of an equimolar amount of bilirubin. The

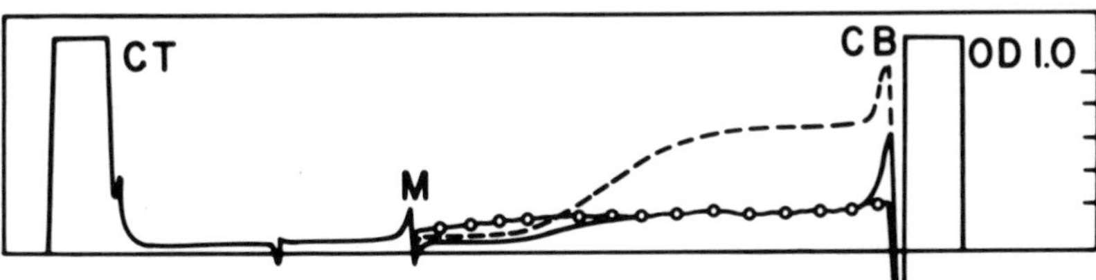

FIGURE 13 Sedimentation–velocity patterns of bilirubin–BSA. CB = cell bottom. The conditions were the same as those described in Figure 12. (a) ○——○, 460 nm, 14-μM bilirubin only, no BSA; (b) ------, 460 nm, [Bilirubin]:[BSA] = 14:7 μM; (c) ————, 375 nm, Same as b. [Reproduced with permission from PJD Publications Ltd., Westbury, N.Y.; from *Research Communications in Chemical Pathology and Pharmacology*, Vol. 6, p. 625 (1973).]

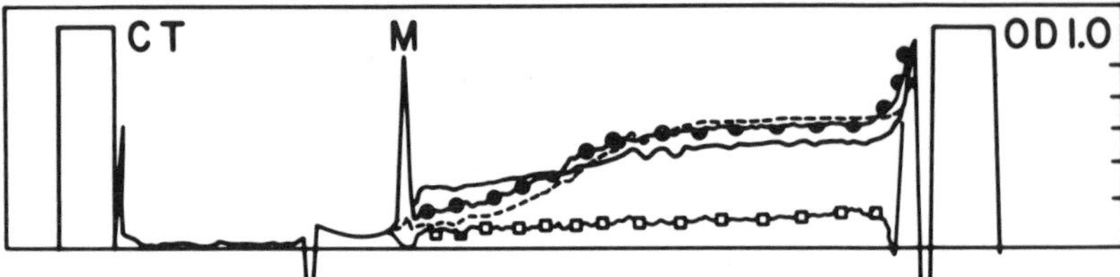

FIGURE 14 Sedimentation–velocity patterns of biliverdin–bilirubin–BSA. [Biliverdin]:[Bilirubin]:[BSA] = 14:14:7 μM. The basal conditions were the same as those described in Figure 12. (a) ———, 375 nm; (b) ●——●, 280 nm; (c) □——□, 650 nm; (d) ------, 460 nm; [Reproduced with permission from PJD Publications Ltd., Westbury, N.Y.; from *Research Communications in Chemical Pathology and Pharmacology*, Vol. 6, p. 625 (1973).]

460-nanometer pattern (dotted line), the scan for bilirubin in the mixture, appeared to be the same as in the bilirubin–BSA system alone [Figure 13(b)]. Thus, it appears that bilirubin–BSA binding is not affected by the presence of biliverdin where the pigments are present in a 1:1:1 proportion (pigments : protein). Although biliverdin does not influence the binding of bilirubin to BSA, this study does not reveal whether bilirubin and biliverdin bind to a common site when each is alone in an equimolar proportion with protein but bind to different sites when mixed.

SOLUBILITY EFFECTS

Another effect became obvious partly by visual observations and partly in some other, more systematic, studies. Definitive concentration studies of this effect have not been done. A mixture of 14-μM biliverdin and 14-μM bilirubin, without BSA, showed some precipitation. Electronic difference spectra of such mixtures showed appreciable suppression of bilirubin absorption in the presence of biliverdin at all pH levels, whether protein was present or not, whereas the absorption of the biliverdin was not affected. This may suggest that biliverdin is affecting the free solubility of bilirubin and that free bilirubin may be salted out of solution by biliverdin, causing changes in bilirubin concentrations. It is doubtful that, in the clinical situation, enough free biliverdin would ever be present in the vascular stream (if it is present at all) to adversely affect small amounts of free bilirubin in the circulation.

Conclusions

The following conclusions can be made: Biliverdin as a free pigment has very little, if any, significant toxicity and is not likely to exist in the bloodstream or in an extravascular tissue location in a high enough concentration to exert any toxic effect or to affect the free solubility of bilirubin. The fact that biliverdin is much more soluble than bilirubin renders it far less likely to cross biological membranes. If biliverdin is a significant photooxidation product *in vivo,* I would think that it should not cause concern. Biliverdin binds to serum albumin but does not adversely affect the protein binding of bilirubin, which is so essential to the maintenance of bilirubin in a nontoxic state.

REFERENCES

1. Blauer, G., D. Harmatz and J. Snir. Optical properties of bilirubin-serum albumin complexes in aqueous solution. I. Dependence on pH. Biochim. Biophys. Acta 278:68–88, 1972.
2. Blauer, G., and T. E. King. Interactions of bilirubin with bovine serum albumin in aqueous solution. J. Biol. Chem. 245:372–381, 1970.
3. Cowger, M. L. Bilirubin encephalopathy, pp. 265–293. In G. E. Gaull, Ed. Biology of Brain Dysfunction. Vol. 2. New York: Plenum Press, 1973.
4. Cowger, M. L., R. P. Igo, and R. F. Labbe. The mechanism of bilirubin toxicity studied with purified respiratory enzyme and tissue culture systems. Biochemistry 4:2763–2770, 1965.
5. Gray, C. H., A. Kulczycka, and D. C. Nicholson. The photodecomposition of bilirubin and other bile pigments. J. Chem. Soc. (Perkin I) 3:288–294, 1972.
6. Gray, C. H., A. Lichtarowicz-Kulczycka, D. C. Nicholson, and Z. Petryka. The chemistry of the bile pigments. Part II. The preparation and spectral properties of biliverdin. J. Chem. Soc. 2264–2268, 1958.
7. Gray, C. H., and D. C. Nicholson. The chemistry of the bile pigments. The structures of stercobilin and *d*-urobilin. J. Chem. Soc. 3085–3099, 1958.
8. Lee, J. J., and M. L. Cowger. Circular dichroism studies of protein-bound biliverdin. Res. Comm. Chem. Pathol. Pharm. 5:505–514, 1973.
9. Lee, J. J., and M. L. Cowger. Conformation of protein-bound bile pigments. Res. Comm. Chem. Pathol. Pharm. 4:121–130, 1972.
10. Lightner, D. A., and G. B. Quistad. Imide products from photo-oxidation of bilirubin and mesobilirubin. Nature (New Biol.) 236:203–205, 1972.
11. Mustafa, M. G., M. L. Cowger, and T. E. King. Effects of bilirubin on mitochondrial reactions. J. Biol. Chem. 244:6403–6414, 1969.
12. Mustafa, M. G., and T. E. King. Binding of bilirubin with lipid: A possible mechanism of its toxic reactions in mitochondria. J. Biol. Chem. 245:1084–1089, 1970.
13. Odell, G. B. Studies in kernicterus. 1. The protein binding of bilirubin. J. Clin. Invest. 38:823–833, 1959.
14. Ostrow, J. D., and R. V. Branham. Photodecomposition of bilirubin and biliverdin *in vitro*. Gastroenterology 58:15–25, 1970.
15. Pressman, B. C. Ionophorous antibiotics as models for biological transport. Fed. Proc. 27:1283–1288, 1968.
16. Wennberg, R. P., and M. L. Cowger. Spectral characteristics of bilirubin–bovine albumin complexes. Clin. Chim. Acta 43:55–64, 1973.

GERARD B. ODELL

Methods for Measurement of the Relative Saturation of Serum Albumin with Bilirubin in the Management of Neonatal Hyperbilirubinemia

In vitro and *in vivo* experimental studies have demonstrated that the cytotoxicity of bilirubin to cells and subcellular organelles occurs if it is freely diffusible in the extracellular fluid to enter cell membranes.[5, 7, 20] The toxicity can be prevented if the extracellular fluid contains albumin and the molar ratio of bilirubin to albumin is below 1;[3, 6, 11, 28] that is, the concentration of diffusible bilirubin is maintained below toxic levels because the affinity of albumin for bilirubin keeps most of the bilirubin in extracellular fluid bound as an albumin–bilirubin ligand.

The association of bilirubin with albumin can be expressed stoichiometrically by mass action formulas:[16, 19]

$$\mathrm{Alb} + \mathrm{B} \leftrightharpoons \mathrm{AlbB} \qquad (1)$$

$$\mathrm{AlbB} + n\mathrm{B} \leftrightharpoons \mathrm{AlbB}_{(n+1)} \qquad (2)$$

The constant governing the unimolar association of bilirubin to albumin has been reported as 10^8 with purified human and 10^6 with bovine albumins (Eq. 1).[2, 8] When the proportion of bilirubin exceeds a 1:1 molar ratio with respect to albumin, secondary sites on the albumin molecule, which have affinity constants in the order of 10^6 (Eq. 2), govern the degree of binding of the additional bilirubin molecules. Given

This study was supported by U.S. Public Health Service grants HD 00091 and HD 02268.

these smaller affinity constants, sufficient bilirubin is dissociated from albumin to cause its diffusible concentration in the aqueous phase of extracellular fluid to be high enough to lead to cytotoxicity. In addition, many other components and properties of extracellular fluid (organic anions, pH, and ionic strength) influence the binding capacity of albumin, for they can alter the primary and secondary binding sites and thereby reduce the ability of albumin to bind bilirubin. It is also suspected that clinical hypoxia, hypoglycemia, and acidosis may make cells more sensitive to the cytotoxicity of bilirubin.

In situations of neonatal hyperbilirubinemia, not all of the high affinity sites in the albumin in the infant's circulation are necessarily available to bind bilirubin. For example, an infant with 3 g/dl of albumin theoretically should not be at risk to bilirubin toxicity until a serum bilirubin concentration of 25 mg/dl is reached, i.e., to the 1:1 molar ratio. However, bilirubin encephalopathy has been reported to occur at concentrations considerably below 25 mg/dl, because endogenous and exogenous substances present in the circulation reduced the binding capacity of albumin for bilirubin.[1, 17, 29, 30] Since both the quality and quantity of albumin in the circulation influence the amount of diffusible bilirubin, a direct measurement of the concentration of diffusible, rather than total, bilirubin would provide a better indicator of the risk of bilirubin toxicity.[18] Unfortunately, the concentration of diffusible bilirubin is so small (less than 0.1 mg/dl) that its quantification is not practicable. Furthermore, as the diffusible bilirubin concentration rises, bilirubin leaves the extracellular fluid, becoming sequestered in cell membranes and intracellular fluid spaces.

Alternative indirect approaches have been developed to measure the diffusible bilirubin concentration; these methods attempt to assess the relative saturation of the albumin carrier with bilirubin. All these saturation tests depend on the implication that, if the albumin is highly saturated with bilirubin, then by Eq. (1) and (2), the concentration of diffusible bilirubin is also elevated and may be at toxic levels.

In principle, four techniques are used to measure the saturation of albumin with bilirubin.

Salicylate Saturation Index[21]

The basis for this test is derived from Eq. (2). If significant amounts of bilirubin are bound to albumin at its lower affinity secondary sites, then some of this bilirubin can be displaced if another organic anion is added to the serum. This occurs when the anion added either binds to albumin at the same binding site as bilirubin or directly influences its binding, and when an association constant for that anion with albumin is of the same order of magnitude as that of bilirubin. Under conditions where the added anion possessing these properties is present, some of the bound bilirubin becomes displaced; i.e., the equilibrium in Eq. (2) is shifted to the left. The test, as run, measures the decrease in absorbance at 460 nm of the protein-bound bilirubin in diluted sera after addition of a standard amount of sodium salicylate as compared to a similarly diluted control sample. The determination, requiring 40 μl of serum, can be made rapidly because equilibrium for the binding of organic anions to albumin is quickly attained.[15]

Experimentally, it is found that only a 14-percent difference in absorbance exists between (1) solutions containing a given concentration of bilirubin that is completely bound to albumin and (2) solutions containing an equal concentration of nonbound (i.e., protein-free) bilirubin. This means, for example, that a 50-percent displacement of previously bound bilirubin by salicylate is reflected only by an 8-percent decrease in the absorbance at 460 nm. To use this test with precision, therefore, one must use calibrated micropipettes and microcuvettes and a spectrophotometer capable of detecting ± 0.002 unit of change in absorbance. In addition, the analysis requires correction of the absorbance at 460 nm for nonbilirubin chromogen in the serum. This correction assumes that bilirubin bound to albumin has the same extinction coefficient in all patients; it necessitates performing an independent chemical determination of the bilirubin concentration so that the absorbance at 460 nm of the serum due to bilirubin can be calculated.

The salicylate saturation test has been used clinically, and its results are reported to reflect with considerable accuracy a significant correlation between the degree of albumin saturation with bilirubin during neonatal hyperbilirubinemia and subsequent cognitive dysfunctions of the central nervous system at 5 years of age.[22]

Dye-Binding Capacity of Jaundiced Serum [10, 24]

The basis for the dye-binding-capacity saturation tests rests on the assumption that the presence of bilirubin bound to albumin diminishes the capacity of the albumin to bind exogenously added dye substances. Originally, the technique was employed to quantitatively measure albumin concentrations in serum by the determination of the change in spectral absorbance of the dye, 2-(4′-hydroxybenzeneazo) benzoic acid (HABA); [26] but, although the dye has a very high affinity for albumin, it was found that the simultaneous presence of bilirubin in the serum interfered with this method for determining albumin and that the method yielded low results. Methyl orange has also been used and was incorporated in many autoanalyzer techniques but, again, in the presence of hyperbilirubinemia, low albumin concentrations were found by this dye-binding assay in contrast to the results of salt or electrophoretic fractionation techniques. The degree of interference to the dye binding was subsequently quantified as a measurement of the relative saturation of the albumin with bilirubin. The technique involves the determination of the amount of HABA bound by a standard pooled serum having a known concentration of albumin containing less than 1.0 mg/dl of bilirubin. The amount bound is compared with that of the test serum. After addition of HABA, the absorbancies of the standard and patient's diluted sera are measured at 510 nm, and the results are expressed as a percentage of HABA bound by the jaundiced serum relative to the standard. This analysis also requires only 40 μl of serum, but the changes in spectral absorbance are greater than with the salicylate method.

This test has been successfully employed in clinical studies to identify infants at risk to bilirubin encephalopathy. A direct comparison of the two techniques on the same serum samples has shown good correlations; that is, high salicylate saturation corresponds to a low HABA binding.[25] The HABA technique is not sensitive to pH (it can be performed at the pH of the patient's serum, whereas the salicylate test does reflect pH influences). However, protein-bound anions other than bilirubin interfere with the HABA binding and, as a consequence, lead to indication of high bilirubin saturations when the actual saturation with bilirubin is considerably lower.

Gel Filtration for Separation of Diffusible and Protein-Bound Bilirubin [9, 12, 14, 32]

As noted above, the direct measurement of diffusible bilirubin in serum might provide a more direct indication of the infant at risk. In these techniques, jaundiced serum is added to a small column of equilibrated Sephadex G-25. An isotonic buffer is then used to filter the sample through the gel matrix. The protein-bound bilirubin is restricted to the void volume of the column, whereas diffusible bilirubin can enter the total volume of the column and is partially adsorbed on the Sephadex particles. After the albumin-bound bilirubin has been eluted, the column is tested for the presence of bilirubin; reagent is added to chemically detect bilirubin, or the bilirubin is eluted from the column with an albumin solution or aqueous alkali. The recovered bilirubin is measured directly from the absorbance of the eluate or after extraction into chloroform.

The eluted protein-free bilirubin is interpreted as diffusible bilirubin. In this technique the Sephadex gel actually binds bilirubin, since the volume of eluant required to recover the bilirubin from the column exceeds the total volume of the column. Thus, the distribution of bilirubin in the column not only represents the protein-bound and the ultrafilterable bilirubin in the native serum but it also reflects the affinity of the Sephadex for bilirubin. As the free bilirubin is adsorbed, dissociation of bilirubin from albumin will occur and enter the column. Because of this adsorption, the column size is important and may explain the variations in diffusible bilirubins reported from different centers using the method. In clinical studies this technique is able to identify infants at risk only after the concentration of diffusible bilirubin becomes high enough to be detected on the column, but it cannot predict relative saturation.

One further adaptation of the column technique has been developed to measure relative saturation.[27] Bilirubin is added to the infant's serum to progressively greater concentrations until protein-free bilirubin is found in the subsequent gel filtrations. The difference between the original concentration of bilirubin in the serum and the final concentration at which protein-free bilirubin first appears in the column reflects the relative saturation. This analysis, however, requires considerably larger serum samples for the serial additions of bilirubin required.

Determination of Concentration of Red-Cell Bilirubin[4]

It has been observed that, in the presence of hyperbilirubinemia,[23, 31] circulating erythrocytes have significant amounts of bilirubin. *In vitro* studies have demonstrated that the molar concentration ratios of bilirubin to albumin can be used to predict how much bilirubin would be sequestered in the red cells when suspended in such solutions.[4, 13] Relatively little bilirubin was recovered from erythrocytes when the molar ratio of bilirubin to albumin in the suspensions was below 1 and crystalline albumin was used. The amount of bilirubin in erythrocytes increased linearly when this ratio was exceeded. However, studies showed that the bilirubin content of circulating erythrocytes from jaundiced infants was considerably more variable than would be predicted from the absolute concentrations of bilirubin and albumin. Such variation should be expected because the circulating albumin contains a variety of anions bound to it that influence its binding affinity for bilirubin.

The determination involves the washing of red cells to free them from trapped plasma and the subsequent elution of the bilirubin from the cells by resuspending them in an albumin solution. The amount of bilirubin eluted is then measured directly.

The determination as reported requires 2 ml of whole blood, which limits its clinical application, but it should be possible to adapt the technique to much smaller volumes by micromethodology. The advantage of this method is that it affords a direct measurement of the amount of bilirubin at the cellular level of the patient with minimal manipulation. The test will identify infants at risk only when the concentration of diffusible bilirubin has become elevated. It does not indicate relative saturation of the serum albumin.

Thus far, all the saturation methods for selecting the infant at risk to bilirubin toxicity have methodological limitations that militate against their application in routine hospital laboratories. Almost all the studies have shown that the relative saturation of circulating albumin with bilirubin in a jaundiced infant can change quite rapidly, and this may not be reflected by much change in the total concentration of serum bilirubin. Saturation tests require serial determinations when the serum bilirubin values are elevated, and this need for repeated determinations requires use of techniques capable of being performed with the small volumes of serum that can be obtained by capillary sampling.

REFERENCES

1. Ackerman, B. D., G. Y. Dyer, and M. M. Leydorf. Hyperbilirubinemia and kernicterus in small premature infants. Pediatrics 45:918–925, 1970.
2. Blauer, G., and T. E. King. Interactions of bilirubin with bovine serum albumin in aqueous solution. J. Biol. Chem. 245:372–381, 1970.
3. Bowen, W. R., E. Porter, and W. J. Waters. The protective action of albumin in bilirubin toxicity in newborn puppies. Am. J. Dis. Child. 98:568, 1959.
4. Bratlid, D. Reserve albumin binding capacity, salicylate saturation index, and red cell binding of bilirubin in neonatal jaundice. Arch. Dis. Child. 48:393–397, 1973.
5. Cowger, M. L., R. P. Igo, and R. F. Labbe. The mechanism of bilirubin toxicity studied with purified respiratory enzyme and tissue culture systems. Biochemistry 4:2763–2770, 1965.
6. Diamond, I., and R. Schmid. Experimental bilirubin encephalopathy. The mode of entry of bilirubin-^{14}C into the central nervous system. J. Clin. Invest. 45:678–689, 1966.
7. Enster, L. The mode of action of bilirubin on mitochondria in kernicterus, p. 174. In A. Sass-Kortsák, Ed. Kernicterus. Toronto: University of Toronto Press, 1961.
8. Jacobsen, J. Binding of bilirubin to human serum albumin—Determination of the dissociation constants. FEBS Lett. 5:112, 1969.
9. Jirsová, V., M. Jirsa, A. Heringová, O. Koldovský, and J. Weirichová. The

use and possible diagnostic significance of Sephadex gel filtration of serum from icteric newborn. Biol. Neonate 11:204–208, 1967.

10. Johnson, L. H., and T. R. Boggs. Failure of exchange transfusion to prevent minimal cerebral damage when employed so as to maintain serum bilirubin concentrations below 18 and 20 mg/100 ml. Pediatr. Res. 4:481, 1970.
11. Johnson, L., M. L. Garcia, E. Figueroa, and F. Sarmiento. Kernicterus in rats lacking glucuronyl transferase. II. Factors which alter bilirubin concentration and frequency of kernicterus. Am. J. Dis. Child. 101:322–349, 1961.
12. Kaufmann, N. A., J. Kapitulnik, and S. H. Blondheim. The adsorption of bilirubin by Sephadex and its relationship to the criteria for exchange transfusion. Pediatrics 44:543–548, 1969.
13. Kaufmann, N. A., A. J. Simcha, and S. H. Blondheim. The uptake of bilirubin by blood cells from plasma and its relationship to the criteria for exchange transfusion. Clin. Sci. 33:201–208, 1967.
14. Keenan, W. J., J. E. Arnold, and J. M. Sutherland. Serum bilirubin binding determined by Sephadex column chromatography. J. Pediatr. 74:813, 1969.
15. Klotz, I. M. Protein interactions, pp. 727–806. In H. Neurath and K. C. Bailey, Eds. The Proteins—Chemistry, Biological Activity, and Methods. Vol. 1, Pt. B. New York: Academic Press, Inc., 1953.
16. Martin, N. H. Preparation and properties of serum and plasma proteins. XXI. Interactions with bilirubin. J. Am. Chem. Soc. 71:1230–1232, 1949.
17. Odell, G. B. Influence of binding on the toxicity of bilirubin. Ann. N.Y. Acad. Sci. 226:225–237, 1973.
18. Odell, G. B. Studies in kernicterus. I. The protein binding of bilirubin. J. Clin. Invest. 38: 823–833, 1959.
19. Odell, G. B. The dissociation of bilirubin from albumin and its clinical implications. J. Pediatr. 55:268–279, 1959.
20. Odell, G. B. The distribution of bilirubin between albumin and mitochondria. J. Pediatr. 68:164–180, 1966.
21. Odell, G. B., S. N. Cohen, and P. C. Kelly. Studies in kernicterus. II. The determination of the saturation of serum albumin with bilirubin. J. Pediatr. 74:214–230, 1969.
22. Odell, G. B., G. N. B. Storey, and L. A. Rosenberg. Studies in kernicterus. III. The saturation of serum proteins with bilirubin during neonatal life and its relationship to brain damage at five years. J. Pediatr. 76:12–21, 1971.
23. Oski, F. A., and J. L. Naiman. Red cell binding of bilirubin. J. Pediatr. 63:1034–1037, 1963.
24. Porter, E. G., and W. J. Waters. A rapid micromethod for measuring the reserve albumin binding capacity in serum from newborn infants with hyperbilirubinemia J. Lab. Clin. Med. 67:660–668, 1966.
25. Priolisi, A., and L. Ziino. Comparative analysis between the reserve albumin-binding capacity (HABA method) and the saturation index of hyperbilirubinemic area. Biol. Neonate 19:258–271, 1971.
26. Rutstein, D. D., E. F. Ingenito, and W. E. Reynolds. The determination of albumin in human blood plasma and serum. A method based on the interaction of albumin with an anionic dye—2-(4′-hydroxybenzeneazo) benzoic acid. J. Clin. Invest. 33:211–221, 1954.
27. Schiff, D., G. Chan, and L. Stern. Sephadex G-25 quantitative estimation of free bilirubin potential in jaundiced newborn infants' sera: A guide to the prevention of kernicterus. J. Lab. Clin. Med. 80:455–462, 1972.

28. Silberberg, D. H., L. Johnson, H. Schutta, and L. Ritter. Effects of photodegradation products of bilirubin on myelinating cerebellum cultures. J. Pediatr. 77:613, 1970.
29. Silverman, W. A., D. H. Andersen, W. A. Blanc, and D. N. Crozier. A difference in mortality rate and incidence of kernicterus among premature infants allotted to two prophylactic antibacterial regimens. Pediatrics 18:614–624, 1956.
30. Stern, L., and R. L. Denton. Kernicterus in small premature infants. Pediatrics 35:483–485, 1965.
31. Watson, D. The absorption of bilirubin by erythrocytes. Clin. Chim. Acta 7:733–734, 1962.
32. Zamet, P., and F. Chunga. Separation by gel filtration and microdetermination of unbound bilirubin. II. Study of sera in icteric newborn infants. Acta Paediatr. Scand. 60:33–38, 1971.

LOIS JOHNSON *and* THOMAS R. BOGGS, JR.

Bilirubin-Dependent Brain Damage: Incidence and Indications for Treatment

As long ago as 1950, Gerver and Day presented evidence to support their postulate that the damage caused by hyperbilirubinemia ranges from obvious kernicterus resulting in death or severe neurologic sequelae to damage so minimal as to be undefinable in any one child.[7] To investigate the latter possibility, they examined the IQ scores of siblings born to couples with Rh incompatibility. They found significantly higher scores ($p<0.001$) among firstborn children who had not been jaundiced in infancy than they found among later-born children who had been jaundiced but, because they had never shown any signs of neurologic impairment, were judged to have escaped damage altogether. In a further study, Day and Haines found the difference between similarly matched sibling pairs to have been decreased, but not eliminated, by treatment with a single exchange transfusion.[4]

In 1967, Vernon investigated the educational handicap of institutionalized "deaf" children, comparing the auditory loss stemming from Rh erythroblastosis during infancy with that resulting from other causes—including congenital deafness.[29] Although the Rh children had more residual hearing than any of the other groups tested, their written

This study was supported by U.S. Public Health Service grants NB05138, NB 06919, and MC R 420022, and by the John H. Hartford Foundation, Inc.

language, speech, and speech-reading did not reflect this advantage. and usable hearing was due to pathology in the areas of auditory perception or integration and sound symbolization. This indicated that damage due to Rh erythroblastosis was broader than generally realized and that more sophisticated psychoaudiometric techniques were needed to properly evaluate its victims.

In the 23 years since Day's first studies, it became standard practice to perform as many exchange transfusions as necessary to keep the concentration of serum bilirubin from exceeding 18–20 mg/100 ml, which Hsia *et al.* found to be the generally accepted threshold for clinical neurologic damage.[8] However, even this more vigorous approach has been found, on closer scrutiny, to offer less than complete protection. For example, a report in 1967 of the results of the 8-month psychological examination among infants enrolled in the Collaborative Project (CORE) demonstrated that motor scores on the Bailey Scale were significantly lower among infants whose concentrations of neonatal serum bilirubin had exceeded 15 mg/100 ml than scores among infants whose bilirubin levels had never exceeded 10 mg/100 ml.[2] This was true even when only infants without evidence of perinatal anoxic insult, as defined by the 5-minute Apgar score, were considered. Additional reports of unsuspected damage soon appeared.[9, 11, 19, 27] One of the most convincing was that of Odell *et al.*, who reported a disturbingly high incidence of central nervous system (CNS) damage, as evidenced by psychometric and neurologic examinations performed at age 5 yr among 32 children in whom the salicylate saturation index and the concentration of serum bilirubin had been measured during the period of neonatal jaundice.[19] Peak concentrations of serum bilirubin ranged from 2 to 31 mg/100 ml. Treatment consisted of one or more exchange transfusions when the bilirubin concentration exceeded 18–20 mg/100 ml. Three of the 18 damaged children had classic neurologic signs of kernicterus, detectable on standard neurologic examination, and 15 had signs of minimal cerebral dysfunction only, the most prominent being impairment of visual perception. In this small number of children, there was no significant correlation of damage with peak concentration of serum bilirubin, although the trend was in the expected direction. However, there was a strong correlation with degree of saturation of the serum proteins with bilirubin. In infants with damage, the mean duration of hyperbilirubinemia in excess of 15 mg/100 ml was longer than in those showing no signs of CNS insult.

Not all recent workers have found a significant incidence of brain damage among infants with concentrations of serum bilirubin below 20 mg/100 ml.[3, 13, 20] Many still consider the 18–20 mg/100 ml level to be the appropriate indication for exchange transfusion. Yet there have been reports of kernicterus among very small, sick infants with concentrations of serum bilirubin of no more than 10–12 mg/100 ml.[6, 26]

Vernon postulated that the discrepancy between the pure tone audiogram

This paper will report data collected in our nurseries during 1965 and 1966 relative to the danger of bilirubin associated with brain damage and the degree to which this damage can be predicted by laboratory measurements and clinical guidelines. Biochemical parameters included estimation of the bilirubin–albumin reserve by the 2-(4′-hydroxybenzeneazo) benzoic acid (HABA) method. CNS function has been estimated by means of follow-up examinations at ages 4 and 7 yr. A preliminary report of the 4-year results has already appeared in abstract form.[11] Analysis of the 7-year results is in progress. Our findings are in essential agreement with those of Odell and of the Collaborative Project.

Material and Methods

The study population consisted of 83 jaundiced infants cared for in the nurseries of Pennsylvania Hospital and Children's Hospital over an 18-month period beginning in late 1964. Treatment consisted of exchange transfusion, sometimes with added albumin, to prevent bilirubin concentrations from rising above 18–20 mg/100 ml. However, outborn infants were often admitted with hyperbilirubinemia in excess of these limits. This study does not include small prematures with respiratory distress syndrome (RDS) and serum bilirubin concentration of about 10 mg/100 ml because the significance of such low bilirubin concentration was not appreciated at the time.

Frequent determinations of serial bilirubin were obtained on all babies. In addition, on all pre-exchange specimens and on as many other specimens as possible, the research laboratory ran the following tests:

- Total serum bilirubin (TSB), direct serum bilirubin, and indirect serum bilirubin (ISB)[15, 31]
- Total serum protein (TP), albumin, and globulin [14]
- Bilirubin–albumin binding reserve by the HABA method (Refs. 10, 23, and L. Johnson, unpublished data)

Most of these specimens were frozen before analysis. Duplicate analyses were run on a representative number at the time of bloodletting and, at a later date, on a deep-frozen aliquot. In nonhemolyzed deep-frozen specimens, the results in the two aliquots were virtually identical.

All follow-up examinations were performed in the Department of Rehabilitation at Children's Hospital. Neurologic examinations were performed under the direction of Dr. Samuel Tucker and included careful scrutiny for the presence of minimal cerebral dysfunction. The psychometric evaluation was developed by Dr. Thomas Atkins and was conducted by him or Mrs. Sandra Wasserstrom. It included the Stanford-Binet test; the Graham Block Sort to assess ability for concept formation; standardized behavioral and social maturity ratings; and assessment of visual perception and fine motor integration by means of the Frostig developmental tests, copy forms, 3-cube pyramid, Wallin Peg Board, and "draw a man." The hearing and language evaluations were conducted by Dr. Richard Winchester and Mrs. Flora Passone, who used a number of techniques originating in Dr. Winchester's audiology laboratory. The techniques permit testing of central auditory perception and central language, including auditory memory and recall and sound symbolization, integration, and response. A more detailed description of the testing program and its significance will be reported elsewhere.

This report considers primarily the findings at age 4 yr in all 83 babies. A subsequent report will be confined to those 67 infants in whom we could be sure that the "binding low" and "bilirubin high" had been measured. Such infants have been arbitrarily defined as those in whom the initial bilirubin binding measurements were made by at least day 3, if term, and day 4, if premature.

Results and Discussion

Tables 1 and 2 describe the study population with respect to sex, Apgar scores, gestational age, incidence of hemolytic disease, and treatment with exchange transfusion. Forty-five of the infants were inborn and 38 outborn. None of the 83 infants had severe apnea and none, after discharge home, had an illness or accident resulting in recognizable anoxic insult to the brain. All the children were from loving and reasonably stable families—largely white and middle class. About 10 percent were black and 25 percent professional.

The incidence of suspect and abnormal ratings (designated together as "not normal") on the speech and hearing, psychometric, and neurologic examinations at age 4 yr is summarized in Table 3.

The greatest incidence of suspect performance was found in the area of visual perception and fine motor integration; 43.5 percent of the children performed in the suspect range on tests assessing this modality. Estimates of the incidence of visual perceptual handicaps in the general population range from 5 to 30 percent.[22, 25] Even the highest estimate is considerably below that found in our study population.

None of the 83 children in the study was found to have peripheral

TABLE 1 Study Population of Children Who Had Neonatal Hyperbilirubinemia: Clinical Diagnosis

Diagnosis	No.
Exchanged	
Idiopathic jaundice	21
Rh-sensitized	30
ABO-sensitized	9
Total	60
No exchange [a]	
Idiopathic jaundice	20
Rh-sensitized	1
ABO-sensitized	2
Total	23
TOTAL	83

[a] The total serum bilirubin did not reach 18 mg/100 ml in the 23 infants who were not treated with exchange transfusion.

sensorineural hearing loss. However, in a disturbingly high number (15.5%), there was evidence of a disorder of central communication functions (Table 3). This figure represents an incidence many times that reported for the population at large, which was estimated in 1969 to be about 2 percent.[28] Even if this is assumed to be an underestimate, the prevalence of such problems in our study population is abnormally high.

Seventeen percent (14 of 83) of the children were rated as less-than-normal on the neurologic examination (Table 3). Eleven had minimal cerebral dysfunction, and three exhibited signs of neurologic damage

TABLE 2 Study Population of Children Who Had Neonatal Hyperbilirubinemia: Sex, Apgar Score, Gestational Age

Apgar Score [a]	No. Babies	No. Males	No. Females
Gestational Age > 37 wk	56	28	28
Apgar > 7	52	25	28
Apgar < 7	4	3	0
Gestational Age < 37 wk	27	14	13
Apgar > 7	19	8	12
Apgar < 7	6	6	1
TOTAL	83	42	41

[a] Nine of the 10 infants with low Apgar scores were males; 8 of the 9 males had suspect ratings on the psychometric examinations at age 4 yr.

TABLE 3 Outcome at Age 4 yr in 83 Infants with Neonatal Jaundice

Test	Not Normal (%)
Psychometric examination	
Overall rating	34.0
Visual perception and fine motor integration	43.5
Neurologic examination	17.0
Minimal cerebral dysfunction only	13.0
Neurologically abnormal	4.0
Peripheral hearing	0.0
Central hearing and central communication [a]	15.5

[a] Includes receptive, integrative, and expressive language and central auditory perception.

(fine and gross motor delay, abnormal reflexes, athetoid movements, mild mental retardation). This is a higher incidence of neurologic deficit than one would anticipate.

Because maleness, immaturity, neonatal anoxia, and prenatal and neonatal complications are known to be associated with a higher incidence of CNS sequelae, we have attempted to assess the way in which these factors are related to the findings reported in Table 3 and to the incidence of high serum bilirubin and low serum binding levels in our study population.

The correlation of gestational age with sex and the major outcome variables is given in Table 4. Premature infants had a higher incidence of an overall suspect rating on the psychometric and neurologic examinations and a lower mean IQ than infants at 37 weeks or more of gestation, but the degree of trend in this small population was not strong enough to be statistically significant. However, there was a significantly higher incidence of bilirubin concentrations of 15 mg/100 ml or more ($p<0.05$) and of HABA-binding levels below 50 percent ($p<0.005$) in prematurely born infants.

Table 5 relates Apgar score to outcome and neonatal variables. There was a significant correlation between Apgar score and sex ($p<0.005$), 9 of the 10 infants with low Apgar scores being male. Low Apgar score also correlated significantly with low binding levels and with an increased incidence of suspect ratings at age 4 yr in both the psychometric and the neurologic test. It did not correlate significantly with bilirubin level, although the trend was in the expected direction.

Sex, regardless of gestational age, also correlated significantly with the major outcome variables (Table 6). However, there was no significant

TABLE 4 Relationship of Gestational Age to Outcome and Various Neonatal Parameters

	Gestational Age (wk)		
	0–36 ($N=27$)	37–40 ($N=56$)	Significance
Suspect [a]			
Neurologic examination (%)	22.0	14.5	Not significant
Psychometric examination (%)	48.0	27.0	Not significant
Mean IQ	106.82	111.53	Not significant
Male (%)	48.0	52.0	Not significant
Binding level ≤ 50% (%)	92.0	48.0	Significant ($p < 0.005$)
Indirect serum bilirubin ≥ 15 mg/100 ml (%)	96.5	74.0	Significant ($p < 0.05$)

[a] Includes abnormal as well as suspect ratings.

TABLE 5 Relationship of Apgar Score to Outcome and Various Neonatal Parameters

	Apgar Score		
	0–6 ($N=10$)	7–10 ($N=73$)	Significance
Mean IQ	100.8	111.3	Significant ($p < 0.05$)
Mean Graham Block score	28.3	35.3	Significant ($p < 0.05$)
Suspect [a]			
Psychometric examination (%)	80.0	27.5	Significant ($p < 0.005$)
Perceptual motor examination (%)	80.0	38.5	Significant ($p < 0.05$)
Neurologic examination (%)	33.5	15.0	Significant ($p < 0.05$)
Male (%)	90.0	45.0	Significant ($p < 0.05$)
Binding level ≤ 50% (%)	100.0	54.5	Significant ($p < 0.05$)
Indirect serum bilirubin ≥ 15 mg/100 ml (%)	100.0	79.5	Not significant

[a] Includes abnormal as well as suspect ratings.

TABLE 6 Relationship of Sex to Outcome and Various Neonatal Parameters

	Male ($N=42$)	Female ($N=41$)	Significance
Mean IQ	105.7	114.5	Significant ($p < 0.01$)
Suspect [a]			
Psychometric examination (%)	52.5	14.5	Significant ($p < 0.001$)
Neurologic examination (%)	26.0	7.0	Significant ($p < 0.05$)
Indirect serum bilirubin (%)			
≥ 20 mg/100 ml	28.5	24.5	Not significant
≥ 15 mg/100 ml	50.0	58.5	Not significant
Binding level ≤ 50% (%)	57.0	51.0	Not significant

[a] Includes abnormal as well as suspect ratings.

correlation of sex either with concentrations of serum bilirubin or with binding level.

Twenty-three of the 83 infants in the study population had what we considered to be significant neonatal complications in addition to hyperbilirubinemia (Table 7). All 10 of the infants with 5-minute Apgar scores of 6 or below had such neonatal complications. Complications

TABLE 7 Outcome of 4-Year Evaluation of All Tests

	Total Number	Ratio Suspect [a] (Percent)	No. Premature	Ratio Suspect [a] (Percent)
Complicated hyperbilirubinemia	23 [b]	17/23 (74.0)	14	10/14 (71.5)
Uncomplicated hyperbilirubinemia	60 [c]	27/60 (45.0)	14	8/14 (57.0)
All infants	83	44/83 (53.0)	28	18/28 (64.5)

[a] In this table a child is counted as suspect if the overall rating on the neurologic, psychometric, or speech and hearing examination was suspect or if the rating on an important group of subtests in one of these examinations was suspect. Examples of important subtests are those pertaining to visual motor functions in the psychometric examination and those pertaining to central auditory perception in the speech and hearing examination.

[b] Ten had low 5-minute Apgar scores and other neonatal complications.

[c] All had 5-minute Apgar scores of 7 or more.

included severe RDS, transient respiratory distress, aspiration pneumonia, sepsis, vomiting, diarrhea, dehydration, and hypoglycemia of 20 mg/100 ml or below. All required specific therapy. In addition, 1 of the 23 had minimal complications that responded to routine nursery care. Fourteen of the 23 were 4–8 weeks premature by gestational age.

Considering all tests, 17 of these 23 infants with *complicated hyperbilirubinemia* (74%) were given suspect ratings on at least one of the three major examinations or on one or more of the subtests assessing the parameters of visual motor perception, central auditory perception, and central language. The three children with neurologic abnormalities fell in this group.

In contrast, 27 of the 60 infants (45%) with *uncomplicated hyperbilirubinemia* were given suspect ratings (Table 7). Fourteen of these 60 infants were premature by gestational age. The population is therefore typical in that these known risk factors were associated with an increased incidence of poor performance in later childhood. But it is important to emphasize that the high incidence of suspect ratings in the infants with uncomplicated hyperbilirubinemia (27 out of 60) suggests that treatment based on the premise that the threshold for damage is 18 mg/100 ml in the premature and 20 mg/100 ml in the term infant does not afford complete protection to the brain. Analysis of the data with respect to peak concentrations of serum bilirubin and bilirubin–albumin-binding reserve supports this proposition and places the threshold for detectable CNS damage at about 15 mg/100 ml even for the term-born infant without other neonatal complications.

Relationship of Hyperbilirubinemia to CNS *Function as Estimated by Psychometric Examination at Age 4 yr*

The relationship between peak concentration of TSB and outcome on the psychometric examination appears in graphic form in Figure 1. While higher concentrations of bilirubin are more common among children rated as suspect or abnormal, this degree of trend in a sample the size of our study population does not reach the level of statistical significance. This is also true when only the indirect-reacting fraction is considered, although the correlation then is better. However, if indirect bilirubin levels are dichotomized, a significant correlation does exist between outcome on the psychometric examination and exposure to hyperbilirubin at the level of 15 mg/100 ml and above (Table 8). The relationship at the 20 mg/100 ml cutoff point, however, is not significant, which points to the considerable risk of brain damage that exists at levels of hyperbilirubinemia between 15 and 20 mg/100 ml. These

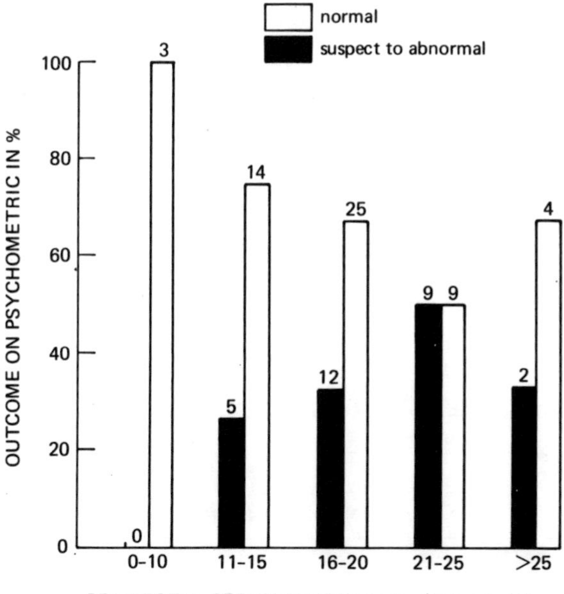

FIGURE 1 Peak TSB concentration versus performance on the psychometric examination. Figures on the horizontal coordinate represent TSB concentration correct to the nearest 1.0 mg/100 ml. Correlation with outcome is not statistically significant but is in the expected direction. In two of the infants, TSB exceeded 25 mg/100 ml, but the indirect-reacting fraction was below 20 mg/100 ml in one and below 15 mg/100 ml in the other. Better correlation is achieved if only indirect bilirubin concentration is considered, but the level of statistical significance is still not reached. NS=not significant.

relationships still hold when only term infants with 5-minute Apgar scores of 7 or more are considered (Table 9) and if all tests, rather than only the psychometric examination, make up the outcome variable.

Intelligence quotients were found to vary inversely with degree of exposure to hyperbilirubinemia (Table 10): A significant lowering of mean IQ scores was found in infants exposed to 4.4, as opposed to 1.7, days of hyperbilirubinemia in excess of 15 mg/100 ml. The mean scores, however, even in infants with the greater degree of exposure, were over

TABLE 8 Relationship of Peak Indirect Serum Bilirubin Concentration to Outcome on the Psychometric Examination at Age 4 yr

Peak ISB [a]	No. Normal	Not Normal No.	Not Normal %	Chi Square
Less than 20 mg/100 ml	44	17	28.0	2.62 (Not significant)
20 mg/100 ml and over	11	11	56.0	
Less than 15 mg/100 ml	14	1	6.5	4.23 ($p < 0.05$)
15 mg/100 ml and over	42	26	38.0	

[a] Indirect serum bilirubin concentration. Concentrations have been corrected to the nearest 0.5 mg/100 ml.

TABLE 9 Incidence of Suspect Ratings at Age 4 yr [a]

Peak ISB [b]	No. Normal	Suspect No.	Suspect %	Chi Square
Less than 15 mg/100 ml	12	2	14.0	$X^2=5.40$ ($p <0.025$)
15 mg/100 ml or more	17	21	55.5	
15–19.5 mg/100 ml	9	11	55.0	Not significant
20 mg/100 ml or more	8	10	55.5	

[a] All infants included in this table had a 5-minute Apgar score of 7 or more and were born at 37 wk of gestation or more.

[b] Indirect serum bilirubin concentration.

[c] In this table a child is counted as suspect if the overall rating on the neurologic, psychometric, or speech and hearing examination was suspect or if the rating on an important group of subtests in one of these examinations was suspect. Examples of important subtests are those pertaining to visual motor functions in the psychometric examination and those pertaining to central auditory perception in the speech and hearing examination.

100 and therefore well within the normal range.* Infants with idiopathic jaundice severe enough to require exchange transfusion were allowed to remain with concentrations of serum bilirubin in excess of 15 mg/100 ml for a longer period than infants with Rh disease, because at that time we were less concerned about jaundice unassociated with hemolytic disease. The lowest mean IQ and the highest incidence of suspect ratings on the psychometric examination were found in these infants at age 4 yr.

* In the CORE project an IQ below 80 is rated as suspect and below 70 is rated as mentally deficient. These are the generally accepted groupings, but for our population the cutoff points are probably too low.

TABLE 10 Relationship of Duration of Hyperbilirubinemia and Type of Jaundice to Mean IQ Score and Rating on Psychometric Examination at Age 4 yr

	Peak Serum Bilirubin < 18–20 mg/ 100 ml [b]	Rh Hemolytic Disease [c]	Idiopathic Jaundice [c]
Number of children	23	30	22
Mean IQ at age 4 yr	114.2 [a]	108.8	103.5 [a]
Children with suspect ratings on psychometric examination (%)	26	30	45
Mean number of days serum bilirubin $\geq$ 15 mg/100 ml	1.7	2.0	4.4

[a] The difference in mean IQ scores is statistically significant ($p < 0.01$).
[b] No exchange.
[c] Exchange transfused.

Relationship of Albumin Binding Reserve to Performance on the Psychometric Examination at Age 4 yr

The correlation between poor performance on the psychometric examination and low binding levels was highly significant (Figure 2), even when the contributions made by anoxia as defined by a low Apgar score and prematurity as defined by gestational age were factored out. Moreover, binding levels correlated significantly with outcome when only males with high Apgars ($N=29$) were considered (Figure 3). The same would almost certainly have been true when only males of 37 weeks or more gestational age and high Apgar scores ($N=23$) were considered, had the numbers been larger (Figure 3). These findings implicate hyperbilirubinemia *per se* as an important cause of CNS insult, additive to, but distinct from, other causes of brain damage. As emphasized by Odell and others and corroborated by these findings, bilirubin-dependent brain damage is more closely related to the degree to which the binding capacity of the serum proteins have been saturated with bilirubin than to the absolute concentration of bilirubin in the serum.[17–19] The threshold for insult to CNS depends on the binding reserve involved, but it appears to be about 15 mg/100 ml of serum bilirubin, a concentration formerly considered safe.

The relationship of binding level to incidence of deficits in visual perception and fine motor integration appears in Figure 4. Correlation at the 0.05 level of significance is present if all babies are considered and

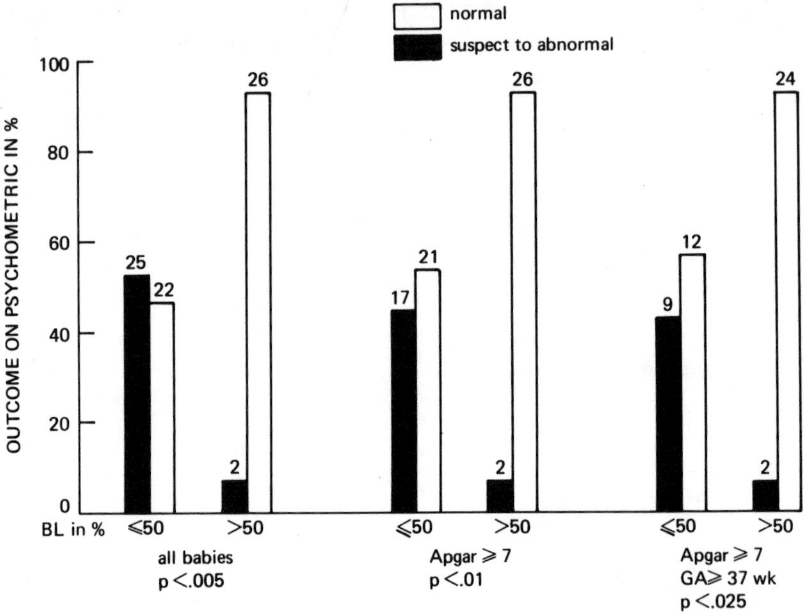

FIGURE 2 Binding level versus performance on the psychometric examination. No binding level measurements were available on 8 of the 83 infants. Ten babies had 5-minute Apgar scores of 6 or less; 27 were premature. The correlation of binding level with outcome persists when the data are controlled for both Apgar score and gestational age (GA).

at the 0.025 level if the 16 less closely monitored infants are omitted (i.e., those infants whose first binding level was obtained after day 3, if term, and day 4, if premature). Deficits in visual perception and fine motor integration are an important cause of learning disability in the early school years. These data suggest that inadequately treated neonatal hyperbilirubinemia is responsible for some of the learning disability found among school-age children.

Others who have investigated the pattern of sequelae following neonatal jaundice [9, 19] and hemolytic disease of the newborn [27] have also found perceptual motor function to be particularly vulnerable to damage. For example, 13 of the 38 children in Hyman's [9] study who were tested in this area were found to have perceptual deficits. Eleven of the 13 had peak concentrations of bilirubin above 15 mg/100 ml, suggesting that the threshold for damage to perceptual motor pathways is about 15 mg/100 ml. However, in her population, 20 mg/100 ml appeared to adequately represent the threshold for other manifestations of CNS damage.

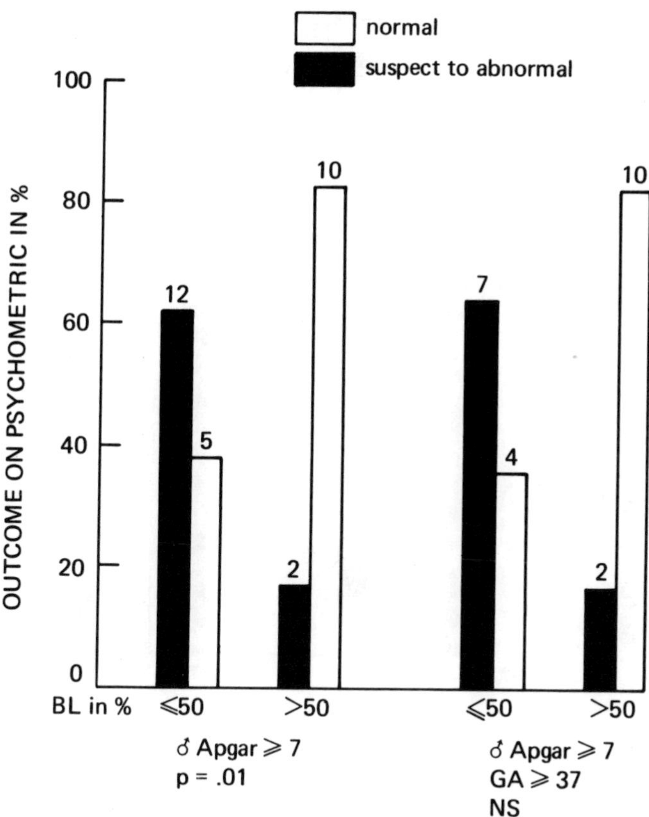

FIGURE 3 Binding level versus performance on the psychometric examination (males only). Binding level predicts outcome on the 4-year psychometric examination in males even when only those with high 5-minute Apgar scores are considered. The trend continues when only high Apgar males born near term are considered but falls below the level of significance when Yates's correction for small numbers is applied. GA=gestational age; NS=not significant.

Duration of Exposure

The duration of exposure to hyperbilirubinemia in excess of 15 mg/100 ml is strongly related to performance on the psychometric examination at age 4 yr. Duration of exposure and binding level were the neonatal parameters that, as individual tests, best predicted the incidence of brain damage in every instance (Figure 5). An infant with an indirect concentration of serum bilirubin of 15 mg/100 ml or more for 0–8 h is

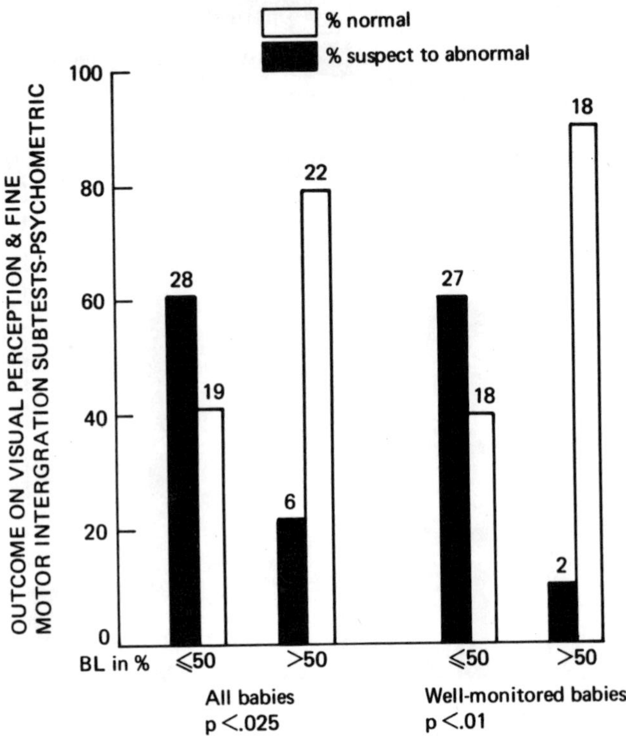

FIGURE 4 Binding level versus performance on the visual perception and fine motor integration subtests of the psychometric examination. The high incidence of visual perceptual deficit in these children correlates well with binding level, especially in the more closely monitored babies.

classified as having 0 days of exposure; one with such a concentration for 9–32 h as having 1 day of exposure; one with such a concentration for 33–56 h as having 2 days of exposure, and so on. On this basis, 1 of 17 infants with 0 days of bilirubin exposure was rated as suspect on the 4-year psychometric examination. In contrast, 26 of 66 infants exposed to such concentrations for more than 8 h were rated as suspect. Three of 29 infants exposed for 1 day or less to this degree of hyperbilirubinemia were rated as suspect as compared with 24 of 54 whose exposure ranged from 2 to 6 or more days. These differences are significant at the 0.025 and 0.005 levels of probability, respectively. Again, damage at a threshold of about 15 mg/100 ml of indirect serum bilirubin is demonstrated.

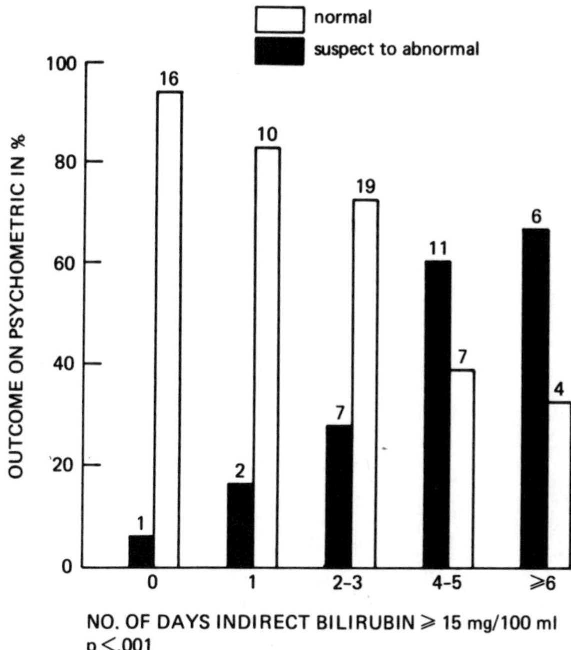

FIGURE 5 Duration of exposure to bilirubin versus performance on the psychometric examination. Concentrations of indirect serum bilirubin are corrected to the nearest 0.5 mg/100 ml. A concentration of 15 mg/100 ml or more for less than 8 h is considered 0 days of exposure. Such a concentration of bilirubin for 8–31 h is considered as 1 day of exposure, 32–56 h as 2 days of exposure, and so on.

Hyperbilirubinemia and CNS *Function as Estimated by the Speech and Hearing Examination at Age 4 yr*

As mentioned previously, no one in our study population was found to have peripheral sensorineural hearing loss, but there was an increased incidence of central communication disorders. Figure 6 relates binding level to outcome on the tests assessing central hearing and central language functions. In this instance a somewhat better correlation was found when binding levels above and below 60 percent were used for comparison. There was a higher incidence of suspect ratings in jaundiced children with binding levels below 60 percent than in those with binding levels above this percentage, but the trend did not reach the level of

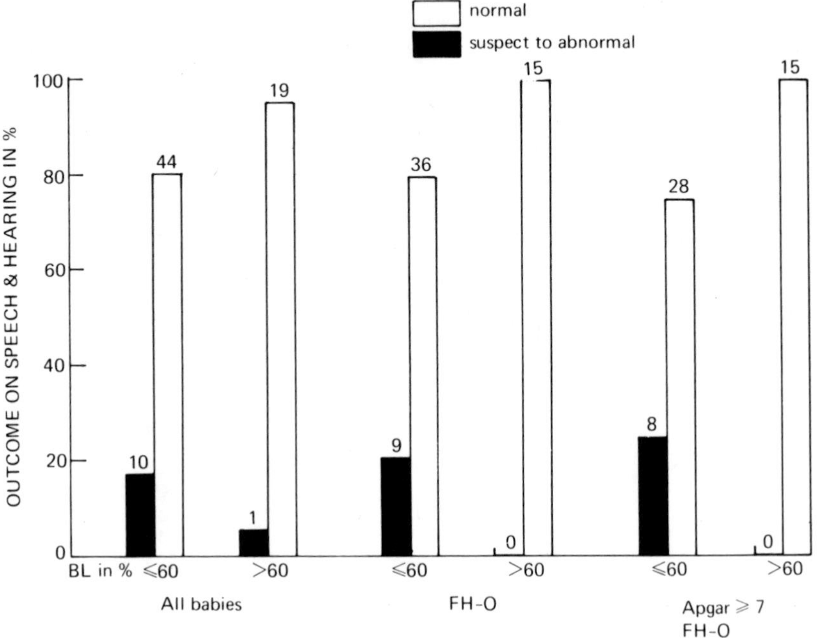

FIGURE 6 Binding level versus performance on the speech and hearing subtests of the psychometric examination. The incidence of language disorder correlates best with binding level when children with a family history of language disorder are excluded, but chi square is still significant only if Yates's correction for small numbers is not applied. (FH-0 = exclusion of infants with a family history of speech disorder.)

statistical significance. If infants with a family history of communication (speech) disorder are excluded and only infants with Apgar scores of 7 and above are considered, the degree of correlation with low binding levels approaches the 0.05 level of probability, even when Yates's correction for small numbers is applied.

As noted earlier, Vernon [29] found evidence of damage to central auditory pathways among a group of institutionalized "deaf" children who had recovered from Rh erythroblastosis. Hyman *et al.*[9] reported a suggestive, but not statistically significant, correlation between deficits in auditory rote memory and high concentrations of serum bilirubin. In contrast to this study, however, Hyman's population also showed an increased incidence of peripheral sensorineural hearing loss.

These findings suggest that the pathways serving the functions of central hearing and central communication are at least as vulnerable to bilirubin insult as are the peripheral nuclei. They also suggest that neonatal hyperbilirubinemia, in spite of treatment with exchange transfusion, is responsible for some of the disorders of language and communication found in the population at large. This may be the case in the absence of associated peripheral hearing loss. Further studies with larger numbers will be required to prove this point.

Hyperbilirubinemia and CNS *Function as Estimated by the Neurologic Examination at Age 4 yr*

The relationship between outcome on the neurologic examination at age 4 yr and bilirubin and binding levels is presented in Table 11. Infants with peak ISB concentrations of 15 mg/100 ml and above have a higher incidence of suspect performance than those with bilirubin concentrations below this level. The trend does not reach statistical significance; however, binding level does correlate significantly with outcome on the neurologic examinations. This is true when all babies are considered ($p<0.025$) and when only babies with a high 5-minute Apgar score are considered ($p<0.05$).

TABLE 11 Outcome of Neurologic Examinations at Age 4 yr [a]

		Not Normal		
	Normal	No.	%	Significance
All babies				
ISB [b] less than 15 mg/100 ml	15	0	0	Not significant
ISB 15 mg/100 ml or more	54	14	19.0	Expected trend
BL [c] over 50%	27	1	3.5	Significant $X^2 = 5.21$
BL 50% or less	34	13	26.5	$p < 0.025$
High Apgar babies				
ISB less than 15 mg/100 ml	15	0	0	Not significant
ISB 15/100 ml or more	47	11	19.0	Expected trend
BL over 50%	27	1	3.5	Significant $X^2 = 4.47$
BL 50% or less	28	10	26.5	$p < 0.05$

[a] All the babies with a low 5-minute Apgar score had binding levels below 50 percent and a peak ISB concentration of 15 mg/100 ml or more. Three of the babies (33%) had suspect to abnormal ratings on the psychometric examination.

[b] Indirect serum bilirubin concentration.

[c] Binding level for HABA dye.

Direct-Reacting Bilirubin

The hyperbilirubinemia of three infants was characterized by a direct-reacting bilirubin glucuronide concentration of over 50 percent. In two of the infants the indirect-reacting fraction was below 15 mg/100 ml. Since HABA binding measurements reflect the presence of bilirubin glucuronide, salicylates, sulfonamides, heme pigments, and free fatty acid—as well as unconjugated bilirubin—the binding level must be interpreted differently when large concentrations of these other protein-bound anions are present. Therefore, binding levels in the three infants just mentioned have been excluded from the analyses presented in this paper.

Bilirubin : Albumin Molar Ratio and Bilirubin : Total Protein Ratio

The bilirubin:albumin molar ratio and the bilirubin:total protein ratio are other potentially valuable indices of risk. As indicated in Figure 7, the bilirubin:albumin molar ratio at the 0.65 dividing line correlates well with outcome on the 4-year psychometric test. However, in contrast to binding level, the correlation falls below the level of statistical significance when the data are controlled for Apgar score. The bilirubin:TP ratio correlates poorly with outcome, which is unfortunate because both total bilirubin and protein are easy to measure. The relative merits of these indices of risk will be considered in more detail elsewhere.

Sex Differences

In sharp contrast to the findings in males, binding level does not accurately predict outcome on the psychometric examination if females alone are considered (Figure 8). In fact, females in comparison with males are remarkably resistant to the toxic effects of hyperbilirubinemia: Only 5 of 41 females, as compared with 22 of 42 males, received less than normal ratings. This is true in spite of the fact that there were a number of instances in females of ISB concentrations over 20 mg/100 ml in association with binding levels below 35 percent and bilirubin:albumin ratios above 0.8. This is a highly interesting phenomenon. Fat has been shown to have a high affinity for bilirubin,[16] one that approaches that of albumin itself. It should therefore provide an effective trap for extravascular bilirubin, effectiveness depending on degree of fatness. These considerations suggest that sex differences in body composition may explain some of the sex differences in outcome that we have observed, since female babies have proportionately more fat, less water, and a smaller mean size than male babies of the same gestational age.[5, 21]

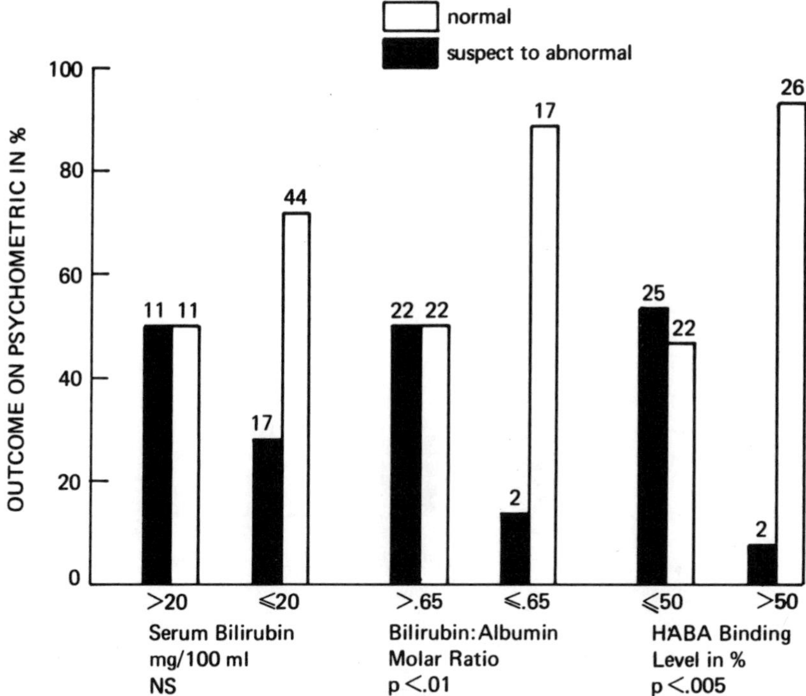

FIGURE 7 ISB, bilirubin : albumin ratio, and binding level versus performance on the psychometric examination. Both the bilirubin : albumin molar ratio and the HABA binding level predict outcome at age 4 yr. In comparison, TSB (correct to the nearest 1.0 mg/100 ml) is a poor indicator of risk.

That extra fat, like extra albumin, actually does offer protection against toxic effects of bilirubin is illustrated by recently completed animal studies in our laboratory. In the Gunn rat we have found a significant reduction of damage to the Purkinje cells in the cerebellar vermis of infant rats suckled on mothers fed a special high-fat breeder chow as compared with infant rats suckled on mothers fed a regular commercial chow (Table 12). Breeder chow babies are noticeably fatter than their regular commercial chow counterparts. Body weight, but not degree of hyperbilirubinemia or concentration of protein in the serum, is associated with the lesser degree of brain damage. The technique of Purkinje cell count as an estimate of brain damage has been described elsewhere.[12, 24]

We have also observed much better breeding and suckling capacities in adult jaundiced females fed breeder chow. On the richer diet, jaun-

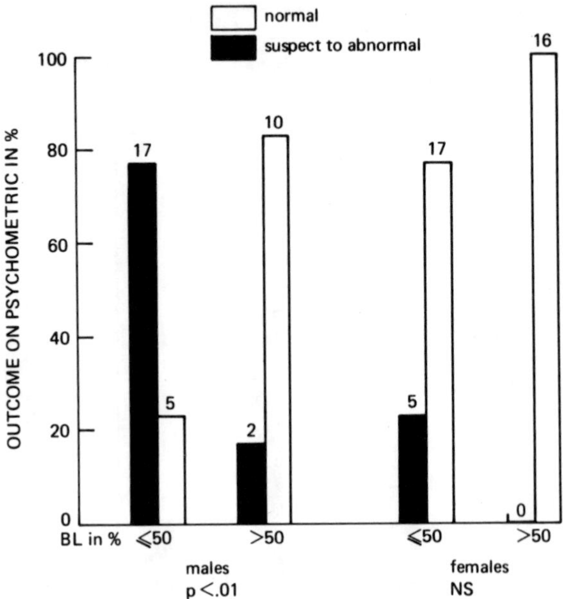

FIGURE 8 Binding level versus performance on the psychometric examination (males and females). Binding level predicts outcome at age 4 yr in males but not in females in spite of similar degrees of exposure to bilirubin. NS=not significant.

TABLE 12 Effect of Diet of Heterozygote Nursing Mother on Suckling Jaundiced Rats, Day 16 (six or seven rats per mother)

Characteristics of Suckling Rats	Regular Commercial Chow 13 males 13 females	Special High-Fat Breeder Chow 9 males 19 females
Mean weight (g)		
Females	36.5	41.5
Males	40.0	47.5
Purkinje cell count, cerebellar vermis [a]		
Mean % normal	38.0	67.0
Mean % abnormal	62.0	33.0
Mean serum bilirubin (mg/100 ml)	13.0	13.5
Mean serum protein (g/100 ml)	5.0	5.0

[a] Clinical neurologic signs are not evident until about 50 percent of the Purkinje cells in such a count are abnormal.[25, 26]

diced female Gunns consistently conceive and carry full-sized litters to term. They can then suckle 6–8 fat offspring to the time of weaning without becoming sick or thin and, after weaning, will promptly conceive again. In contrast, female jaundiced Gunns fed regular commercial chow conceive irregularly and reabsorb most of the products of conception that do occur. The babies are scrawny, and most of them soon die. Occasionally one or two from such a litter survive, exhibiting severe neurologic (kernicteric) damage, and the mother becomes thin and exhausted.

Differences in quantity of body fat secondary to increased caloric (fat) intake, rather than differences in nutrition related to specific factors, such as vitamin E intake, seem to explain these striking differences.

It is important to remember, however, that an alternative explanation for some of the poor performance of boys as compared with that of girls may lie in the difference in maturation rate of the sexes. This difference would give 4-year-old girls a temporary advantage over 4-year-old boys if both are judged by the same age norms. Preliminary analysis of the results of the 7-year follow-up suggests that this is the case. There is a relatively improved performance in boys and a less good performance in girls at age 7 yr, especially among those with low bindings and high bilirubins. Nevertheless, the higher incidence of suspect ratings among males persists at the 7-year follow-up. These findings are illustrated in Table 13, which considers only infants with uncomplicated hyperbilirubinemia in the 15.0–19.5 mg/100 ml range. Seventy-five percent of the males, as compared with 17 percent of the females, received suspect ratings in some area of the 4-year evaluation—a significant difference at the 0.05 level of probability. At the 7-year evaluation, 55 percent of the males—as compared with 25 percent of the females—received suspect ratings, which represents a considerable improvement among males and suggests that, at age 4 yr, males and females should be judged by different norms. Although the difference between the sexes is not statistically significant (because of the small numbers involved), it is impressive and is in harmony with the generally accepted greater vulnerability of the infant male at a later age.

Combined Risk Indices and Need for Treatment

Tables 14 and 15 show the effect of combining risk indices. Table 14 upper third compares high-risk infants (those with "high" bilirubin and "low" binding levels with low-risk infants (those with "low" bilirubin and "high" binding levels) with respect to outcome at age 4 yr. Suspect ratings in the 4-year follow-up examination (one aspect or more) were given to 63.5 percent of the infants in the high-risk group; in contrast, only 14.5 percent in the low-risk group received such ratings—an inci-

TABLE 13 Infants with Uncomplicated Hyperbilirubinemia: Incidence of Suspect Ratings in 4- and 7-Year Follow-ups, All Tests [a]

	Ratio Suspect at Age 4 yr [b]		Ratio Suspect at Age 7 yr [b]	
	Females	Males	Females	Males
Birth weight over 2500 g Peak ISB [c] 14.8–19.7 mg/100 ml	2/9	8/11	1/7	5/10
Birth weight 1800–2500 g Peak ISB 14.8–18.2 mg/100 ml	1/2	1/1	1/1	1/1
Both weight groups	3/11 (27%)	9/12 (75%)	2/8 (25%)	6/11 (55%)
Overall	12/23 (52%)		8/19 (42%)	

[a] This table considers outcome among infants with uncomplicated hyperbilirubinemia whose peak ISB concentrations reached 15 mg/100 ml or more but remained below the 18–20 mg/100 ml level that was recommended for exchange transfusion at the time. "Infants with uncomplicated hyperbilirubinemia" includes vigorous, nonedematous infants with hemolytic jaundice whose cord hemoglobin was 12 g/100 ml or more. It excludes infants with jaundice complicated by other neonatal problems, including relatively minor ones, such as a 5-minute Apgar score of 6 or less and weight loss approaching 10 percent of birth weight.

[b] There is a significant sex difference in incidence of suspect ratings at 4 years of age ($p < 0.05$) but not at 7 years of age.

[c] Indirect serum bilirubin concentration.

dence that probably represents a background of morbidity with respect to CNS function, entirely unrelated to bilirubin. Correlation obtained with this combined risk index is somewhat better than that obtained when binding level alone is considered ($p<0.005$). The lower two thirds of Table 14 suggest that ISB concentrations of over 15 mg/100 ml are not safe unless the HABA binding reserve exceeds 60 percent.

Table 15 shows the added contribution of sex and neonatal complications to the high-risk category. In this maximum-risk group, consisting of males with high bilirubins, low bindings, and other neonatal complications, there was a 100-percent incidence of suspect ratings on the 4-year follow-up. Obviously, all these high-risk groups need prompt treatment.

Between these two extremes lies a group of infants with binding level above 50 percent and ISB of 15 mg/100 ml or more (Table 14). If the binding level is as high as 60 percent, there seems to be little bilirubin-associated risk since the incidence of suspect ratings in this group (12.5%) is virtually the same as that found in the low-risk babies (14.5%). But if the binding level lies in the 50–60 percent range with

TABLE 14 Combined Risk Indices: Relationship to Outcome at Age 4 yr, All Tests

Test Characteristics	No. Normal	Suspect [a] No.	Suspect [a] %	Significance
BL [b] 50% or less ISB [c] 15 mg/100 ml or more	17	30	63.5	$X^2=8.72$
BL over 50% ISB less than 15 mg/100 ml	12	2	14.5	$p < 0.005$
BL 50% or less ISB 15 mg/100 ml or more	17	30	63.5	Not significant
BL 50% or more ISB 15 mg/100 ml or more	6	9	40.0	Expected trend
BL 60% or less ISB 15 mg/100 ml or more	19	35	65.0	$X^2=5.83$
BL 60% or more ISB 15 mg/100 ml or more	7	1	12.5	$p < 0.025$

[a] In this table a child is counted as suspect if the overall rating on the neurologic, psychometric, or speech and hearing examination was suspect or if the rating on an important group of subtests in one of these examinations was suspect. Examples of important subtests are those pertaining to visual motor functions in the psychometric examination and those pertaining to central auditory perception in the speech and hearing examination.

[b] Binding level for HABA dye.

[c] Indirect serum bilirubin concentration.

this degree of jaundice, a 40-percent incidence of suspect ratings still occurs and treatment of some sort is indicated.

With respect to HABA binding levels of more than 60 percent, it should be noted that such a binding reserve is practically never seen when the test is accurately run with an ISB concentration in the approximate amount of 18 mg/100 ml unless considerable parenteral albumin has been previously administered. Since the HABA-binding measurement is an indirect estimate of the tendency of bilirubin to migrate to extravascular binding sites, the actual amount of bilirubin that leaves the bloodstream at a given level of binding reserve will depend on the concentration of bilirubin in the serum, as well as on such important variables as acid base balance and osmolarity. For these reasons, *binding levels should never be interpreted out of context,* and it is probably unwise to withhold exchange transfusion, especially from male infants, if the ISB ex-

TABLE 15 Outcome at 4 Years of Age: Incidence of Suspect Ratings, All Tests [a]

Test Characteristics	Ratio (Percent) of Children Suspect		
	Females	Males and Females	Males
ISB [b] 15 mg/100 ml or less BL [c] over 50%	1/7 (14.0)	2/12 (16.5)	1/5 (20.0)
ISB 15 mg/100 ml or less BL 50% or less	—	—	—
ISB 15 mg/100 ml or more BL over 50%	3/8 (37.5)	6/15 (40.0)	3/7 (42.5)
ISB 15 mg/100 ml All binding levels	12/30 (40.0)	34/62 (55.0)	22/32 (69.0)
BL 50% or less All bilirubin levels	9/22 (41.0)	30/47 (63.0)	21/25 (84.0)
Infants with other complications [d] ISB 15 mg/100 ml or more BL 50% or less	2/7 (28.5)	14/19 (73.5)	12/12 (100.0)

[a] In this table a child is counted as suspect if the overall rating on the neurologic, psychometric, or speech and hearing examination was suspect or if the rating on an important group of subtests in one of these examinations was suspect. Examples of important subtests are those pertaining to visual motor functions in the psychometric examination and those pertaining to central auditory perception in the speech and hearing examination.

[b] Indirect serum bilirubin.

[c] Binding level for HABA dye.

[d] Twelve of these 19 infants were premature by weight; 14 were premature by gestational age.

ceeds 20 mg/100 ml, regardless of binding levels. At the other extreme, sick premature infants should be treated if the ISB reaches 10 mg/100 ml. Binding levels in such infants are uniformly low, however, and in themselves suggest the need for treatment regardless of the "low" concentrations of bilirubin in the serum.

Concluding Comments

We by no means anticipated finding such a high incidence of damage among infants whose concentrations of serum bilirubin had been maintained, by and large, within what were then considered safe limits

(1965–1966). Damage, we had thought, would be confined to those few infants whose hyperbilirubinemia was complicated by other problems, such as acidosis and anoxia. And we had looked forward to finding a sizable number of term infants with uncomplicated hyperbilirubinemia who would prove not to be at risk in spite of concentrations of serum bilirubin of 18–20 mg/100 ml. Instead, we found the distressingly high sequelae rate at the lower concentrations reported here.

It may be argued that exchange transfusion, in inexperienced hands, is too dangerous a treatment if the risk associated with nontreatment is, much of the time, subtle and limited in degree. But it must be admitted that the risk is negligible where the treatment is in experienced hands [1, 30] and that learning disorders associated with minimal brain damage are significant handicaps.[22, 25]

The need for safe, simple, effective modes of therapy to supplement treatment with exchange transfusion in the management of neonatal jaundice is apparent. A major reason for the need is that accurate estimates of binding reserve are usually unavailable to clinicians. Since phototherapy gives promise of fulfilling the requirements, it deserves to be subjected to rigorous controlled testing with all possible speed. This testing should include a thorough, long-term follow-up.

Acknowledgments

The authors wish to thank Mr. Tony Mignano, Miss Marcia Gluyas, and Miss Sandra Valenta for technical assistance; Mrs. Betty Lamplugh for research assistance; Mrs. Sharon Oaks, Mrs. Susan Stapleton, and Mrs. Dorothy Neff for secretarial help; Dr. Michael Sheff and Dr. Alan Goldman for consultation and advice; and the nursing and resident staff for help in collecting specimens and in implementing the study design.

REFERENCES

1. Boggs, T. R., Jr. Comment on the pitfall of overuse of exchange transfusion for treating neonatal hyperbilirubinemia. Pediatr. Clin. North Am., 12:99–100, 1965.
2. Boggs, T. R., Jr., J. B. Hardy, and T. M. Frazier. Correlation of neonatal serum total bilirubin concentrations and developmental status at age eight months. J. Pediatr. 71:553–560, 1967.
3. Culley, P., J. Powell, J. Waterhouse, and B. Wood. Sequelae of neonatal jaundice. Br. Med. J. 3:383–386, 1970.
4. Day, R. L., and M. S. Haines. Intelligence quotients of children recovered from erythroblastosis fetalis since the introduction of exchange transfusion. Pediatrics 13:333–337, 1954.

5. Fomon, S. J. Body composition of the male reference infant during the first year of life. Borden Award Address, October 1966. Pediatrics 40:863–870, 1967.
6. Gartner, L. M., R. N. Snyder, R. S. Chabon, and J. Bernstein. Kernicterus: High incidence in premature infants with low serum bilirubin concentrations. Pediatrics 45:906–917, 1970.
7. Gerver, J. M., and R. L. Day. Intelligence quotients of children who have recovered from erythroblastosis fetalis. J. Pediatr. 36:342–348, 1950.
8. Hsia, D. Y.-Y., F. H. Allen, Jr., S. S. Gellis, and L. K. Diamond. Erythroblastosis fetalis. Studies of serum bilirubin in relation to kernicterus. N. Engl. J. Med. 247:668–671, 1952.
9. Hyman, C. B., J. Keaster, V. Hanson, I. Harris, R. Sedgwick, H. Wursten, and A. R. Wright. CNS abnormalities after neonatal hemolytic disease or hyperbilirubinemia. A prospective study of 405 patients. Am. J. Dis. Child. 117:395–405, 1969.
10. Johnson, L., and T. Boggs. An Estimate of the Kernicteric Potential of Jaundiced Sera. American Pediatric Society 67th Meeting, Proceedings and Abstracts, 1966.
11. Johnson, L. H., and T. R. Boggs. Failure of exchange transfusion to prevent minimal cerebral damage when employed so as to maintain serum bilirubin concentrations below 18 and 20 mg/100 ml. Pediatr. Res. 4:481, 1970.
12. Johnson, L., and H. S. Schutta. Quantitative assessment of the effects of light treatment in infant Gunn rats. Birth Defects 6:114–118, 1970.
13. Johnston, W. H., V. Angara, R. Baumal, N. A. Hawke, R. H. Johnson, S. Keet, and M. Wood. Erythroblastosis fetalis and hyperbilirubinemia—a five-year follow-up with neurological, psychological, and audiological evaluation. Pediatrics 39:88–92, 1967.
14. Kingsley, G. R. The determination of serum total protein, albumin, and globulin by the biuret reaction. J. Biol. Chem. 131:197–200, 1939.
15. Malloy, H. T., and K. A. Evelyn. The determination of bilirubin with the photoelectric colorimeter. J. Biol. Chem. 119:481–490, 1937.
16. Mustafa, M. G., and T. E. King. Binding of bilirubin with lipid: A possible mechanism of its toxic reactions in mitochondria. J. Biol. Chem. 245:1084–1089, 1970.
17. Odell, G. B. The distribution and toxicity of bilirubin. E. Mead Johnson Address, 1969. Pediatrics 46:16–24, 1970.
18. Odell, G. B., S. N. Cohen, and P. C. Kelly. Studies in kernicterus. II. The determination of the saturation of serum albumin with bilirubin. J. Pediatr. 74:214–230, 1969.
19. Odell, G. B., G. N. B. Storey, and L. A. Rosenberg. Studies in kernicterus. III. The saturation of serum proteins with bilirubin during neonatal life and its relationship to brain damage at five years. J. Pediatr. 76:12–21, 1971.
20. Ose, T., T. Tsuruhara, M. Araki, T. Hanaoka, and O. B. Bush. Follow-up study of exchange transfusion for hyperbilirubinemia in infants in Japan. Pediatrics 40:196–201, 1967.
21. Owen, G. M., R. L. Jensen, and S. J. Fomon. Sex-related difference in total body water and exchangeable chloride during infancy. J. Pediatr. 60:858–868, 1962.
22. Paine, R. S. Syndromes of "minimal cerebral damage". Pediatr. Clin. North Am. 15:779–801, 1968.

23. Porter, E. G., and W. J. Waters. A rapid micromethod for measuring the reserve albumin binding capacity in serum from newborn infants with hyperbilirubinemia. J. Lab. Clin. Med. 67:660–668, 1966.
24. Schutta, H. S., and L. Johnson. Bilirubin encephalopathy in the Gunn rat: A fine structure study of the cerebellar cortex. J. Neuropathol. Exp. Neurol. 26:377–396, 1967.
25. Slingerland, B. H. Teacher's Manual to Accompany Screenings Test for Identifying Children with Specific Language Disability. (Rev. ed.) Cambridge, Mass.: Educator's Publishing Service, Inc., 1969.
26. Stern, L., and R. L. Denton. Kernicterus in small premature infants. Pediatrics 35:483–485, 1965.
27. Stewart, R. R., W. Walker, and R. D. Savage. A developmental study of cognitive and personality characteristics associated with haemolytic disease of the newborn. Develop. Med. Child. Neurol. 12:16–26, 1970.
28. U.S. Department of Health, Education, and Welfare, National Institutes of Health, National Institute of Neurological Diseases and Stroke, National Advisory Neurological Diseases and Stroke Council. Human Communication and its Disorder—An Overview. Bethesda, Md.: U.S. Dept. Health, Education, and Welfare, 1969. 176 pp.
29. Vernon, McC. V. Rh factor and deafness: The problem, its psychological, physical, and educational manifestations. Except. Child. 34:5–12, 1967.
30. Weldon, V. V., and G. B. Odell. Mortality risk of exchange transfusion. Pediatrics 41:797–801, 1968.
31. White, D., G. A. Haidar, and J. G. Reinhold. Spectrophotometric measurement of bilirubin concentrations in the serum of the newborn by the use of a microcapillary method. Clin. Chem. 4:211–222, 1958.

PAUL Y. K. WU

Immediate and Long-Term Effects of Phototherapy on Preterm Infants

The effectiveness of phototherapy in the prevention and control of hyperbilirubinemia in the newborn nurseries has been demonstrated in a number of controlled studies. Several of these studies were reviewed by Lucey.[8] Nevertheless, many questions related to this form of therapy remain unanswered. The most appropriate schedule of treatment has not been thoroughly investigated, nor have the immediate and long-term effects of prolonged phototherapy of the neonate been documented. In view of this, several studies were conducted from 1970 up to the present time at our medical center. Their purposes were to determine the effectiveness of intermittent phototherapy in preventing hyperbilirubinemia in preterm infants, to compare the effectiveness of continuous versus intermittent phototherapy, to determine whether there are any short- or long-term effects on growth and development of infants exposed to phototherapy, and to study some of the side effects of phototherapy on the neonate.

The photoenergy source for these studies consisted of a bank of 10 preheat trigger, 20-watt, daylight fluorescent lamps. Irradiance measure-

This study was supported by grants from The Birely Foundation, Mead Johnson Co., and Professional Staff Association of the Los Angeles County-USC Medical Center and by Grant No. 5S01 RR 05466–05 from the U.S. Department of Health, Education, and Welfare.

TABLE 1 Weight Changes on Seventh Day

	Weight Gain [a]		Weight Loss [a]	
Group	Amount (g)	% Infants	Amount (g)	% Infants
Control (C)	97.3 ± 76.4	80.0	83.3 ± 57.9	20.0
Continuous (A)	90.9 ± 74.5	44.0	85.0 ± 61.4	66.0
Intermittent (B)	105.3 ± 77.7	57.6	52.7 ± 45.1	42.4

[a] Mean ± SD.

ments, taken with filters and the Kendall Mark IV Radiometer and conducted in an isolette incubator at the infant position, under plexiglass cover, were 0.245 and 0.277 mW/cm^2 for wavebands of 420–460 nm and 460–500 nm, respectively.* Visible light intensity as measured by a GE photometer was 450–500 ft-c at the infant level.

Growth and Neurological Responses

In order to study the relative effectiveness of intermittent versus continuous phototherapy and the immediate effect of such therapy on growth and neurological responses, 120 infants (birth weight, 1250–2000 g) were placed randomly in three groups at 24 hours of age. Group A (40) received continuous phototherapy for 5 days; Group B (40) received intermittent phototherapy (12 h on and 12 h off) for 5 days; Group C (40) were used as controls and did not receive any phototherapy. The mean birth weight, gestational age, and fluid and caloric intake were comparable in the three groups. The naked infants were nursed in an incubator; their skin temperature was maintained at 36.5–37 °C either with a servocontrol or by regulating incubator temperature.

At the end of the seventh day, 44 percent of Group A, 57.6 percent of Group B, and 80 percent of Group C had regained their birth weight (Table 1). Although the total number of infants in Group B who regained and exceeded their birth weight was less than in Group C, in those that did gain, the mean-weight gain was greater than that of the infants in Group C.

Similar, but less marked, changes were seen in length and head circumference (Tables 2 and 3). Groups A and B had greater increases in

* Measurements were made in conjunction with Mr. Martin Berdahl, thermodynamicist, Space Instruments Section of the Jet Propulsion Laboratory, California Institute of Technology, Pasadena.

TABLE 2 Changes in Body Length

Group	Changes in Body Length, by Week (cm) [a]			
	1	2	3	4
Control (C)	1.2 ± 0.9	0.6 ± 0.5	0.6 ± 0.5	0.8 ± 0.7
Continuous (A)	0.8 ± 0.7	0.8 ± 0.6	0.9 ± 0.7	0.7 ± 0.6
Intermittent (B)	0.9 ± 0.7	0.8 ± 0.6	0.7 ± 0.5	0.5 ± 0.4

[a] Mean ± SD.

weight and length than Group C during the second and third postnatal weeks (Table 4). Increase in head circumference was greater in Group A than in Groups B and C in the second week (Table 3). No significant differences were observed in mean increments in body weight, length, and head circumference in the three groups during the third and fourth weeks.

Moro, sucking reflex, muscle tone, and traction responses were scored weekly as indices of neurological response. In general, Group C appeared to score slightly better than A and B on the seventh day (Table 5). There were no differences in the mean scores in all the groups in subsequent weeks.

The mean levels of serum bilirubin are shown in Table 6. The data suggest decrease in growth and poorer neurological response during continuous phototherapy with subsequent catch-up during the second and third weeks. Differences were less marked between infants on intermittent phototherapy and the controls. These observed differences are intriguing. Observations on stunting of growth in animals by visible radiation are relatively few. G. D. Bruckner *et al.*—cited by Hollwich [3]—studied the effect of varying amounts of radiant energy within the visible

TABLE 3 Changes in Head Circumference

Group	Changes in Head Circumference, by Week (cm) [a]			
	1	2	3	4
Control (C)	0.5 ± 0.3	0.7 ± 0.4	0.9 ± 0.4	0.9 ± 0.5
Continuous (A)	0.4 ± 0.4	0.9 ± 0.4	0.8 ± 0.5	1.1 ± 0.4
Intermittent (B)	0.7 ± 0.6	0.6 ± 0.3	1.0 ± 0.5	0.9 ± 0.6

[a] Mean ± SD.

TABLE 4 Weight Gain in Subsequent Weeks

	Weight Gain, by Week (g) [a]		
Group	2	3	4
Control (C)	139.0 ± 69.8	184.5 ± 55.5	193.6 ± 82.3
Continuous (A)	162.4 ± 62.3 [b]	225.3 ± 62.5 [b]	195.5 ± 74.2
Intermittent (B)	161.7 ± 82.7 [b]	168.1 ± 103.9	179.4 ± 63.1

[a] Mean ± SD.
[b] $p < 0.05$.

light on New Hampshire chickens and found that the group receiving the maximum exposure had poorer weight gain, were less active, and had a higher mortality. Wu *et al.*[22] recently reported similar findings in newborn Sprague–Dawley rats and rabbits. The unfavorable influence of light on growth has also been reported in other species.[5, 11, 13, 15, 17–19] In addition, it has been shown in recent years that DNA synthesis in mammalian tissues, as well at mitotic activity, is characterized by regular diurnal rhythm.[1, 9, 10, 12, 16] Whether continuous exposure to light energy for several days can interfere with the diurnal rhythm in the human neonate is not clear. Conceivably, as Wurtman had indicated,[23] nerve impulses produced by exposure to light may stimulate neuroendocrine-transducers (e.g., the pineal gland and neurosecretory hypothalamus region) to produce hormones that may affect the functions of target organs, and this in turn may affect body metabolism.

It appears that some of the side effects of phototherapy (e.g., changes in blood flow, body temperature, and insensible water loss) may also influence the metabolic rate in neonates on phototherapy. Such changes may contribute to the differences in weight gain and growth.

TABLE 5 Neurological Responses on Seventh Day

	Neurological Response Score [a]			
Group	Tone	Moro	Suck	Traction
Control (C)	2.1 ± 0.7	2.7 ± 0.7 [b]	3.3 ± 1.0 [b]	2.0 ± 0.8
Continuous (A)	2.1 ± 0.9	2.3 ± 0.8	2.8 ± 1.1	2.0 ± 0.9
Intermittent (B)	2.1 ± 0.8	2.5 ± 0.6	2.9 ± 1.1	2.1 ± 0.8

[a] Score: Absent, 0; poor, 1; fair, 2; good, 3; increased, 4.
[b] $p < 0.05$.

TABLE 6 Serum Bilirubin Mean Levels During Phototherapy

Group	Serum Bilirubin by Day of Phototherapy (mg/100 ml) [a]						
	1	2	3	4	5	6	7
Control (C)							
a.m.	7.0 ± 2.5	8.3 ± 2.7	9.4 ± 3.5	8.7 ± 3.9	8.4 ± 4.0	6.4 ± 2.4	5.9 ± 2.8
p.m.	7.7 ± 2.6	8.3 ± 2.7	9.4 ± 3.5	7.9 ± 3.3	6.7 ± 3.5	6.1 ± 2.1	4.9 ± 2.1
Continuous (A)							
a.m.	7.0 ± 2.0	6.7 ± 2.3	6.3 ± 2.3	5.2 ± 1.8	4.8 ± 2.3	4.4 ± 1.8	5.0 ± 2.3
p.m.	6.4 ± 1.9	5.8 ± 2.0	4.9 ± 1.5	4.6 ± 1.5	4.8 ± 2.3	4.4 ± 1.7	4.6 ± 2.1
Intermittent (B)							
a.m.	7.3 ± 2.0	7.9 ± 2.6	7.0 ± 2.4	6.9 ± 2.6	6.0 ± 2.7	5.4 ± 2.5	5.4 ± 2.4
p.m.	6.6 ± 1.8	6.3 ± 1.9	6.6 ± 2.8	5.8 ± 2.5	5.2 ± 2.3	4.8 ± 2.1	4.7 ± 2.3

[a] Mean ± SD.

TABLE 7 Changes in Blood Flow, Temperature, and Rates of Respiration and Heartbeat with Phototherapy (First Study)

	Prephototherapy ($\overline{m} \pm 1$ SD)	Phototherapy ($\overline{m} \pm 1$ SD)	"t" Test
Blood flow (ml/100 ml tissue/min)			
Total	9.98 ± 1.40	21.73 ± 5.18	$p < 0.01$
Muscle	5.58 ± 1.22	7.43 ± 1.60	$p < 0.02$
Skin	4.40 ± 1.0	14.31 ± 4.92	$p < 0.05$
Temperature (°C)			
Skin	36.1 ± 0.6	36.7 ± 0.8	$p < 0.05$
Rectal	36.4 ± 0.7	36.7 ± 0.8	Not significant
Incubator	33.9 ± 1.4	35.4 ± 1.6	$p < 0.05$
Respiration (rate/min)	47.0 ± 9.0	62.0 ± 11.0	$p < 0.01$
Heartbeat (rate/min)	143.0 ± 3.0	162.0 ± 10.0	$p < 0.01$

SOURCE: Data from Wu *et al.*[21]

Blood Flow

The phenomenon of vasodilatation and erythema in the skin on exposure to ultraviolet (UV) radiation is well known.[6, 7] Radiant energy from phototherapy lamps with an intervening plexiglass cover almost completely eliminates radiation in the short UV wavelengths;[14, 24] however, a significant proportion of the long UV and near UV wavelengths do pass through the plexiglass cover.* To what extent irradiation from phototherapy lamps will influence peripheral circulation is not known. In order to study this, the electrocapacitance plethysmograph with local counter pressure[4] was adapted for measuring total blood flow and blood flow through the skin and muscle in the calf. Twenty icteric preterm infants (mean birth weight, 1691 g; mean postnatal age, 5 days) were studied. Two sets of blood-flow measurements were recorded from each infant, once before and once during phototherapy. The infants were divided for two studies. In the first study, involving 10 infants, no attempt was made to alter the prephototherapy incubator settings. The results indicate that, during phototherapy, total blood flow increased by a mean of 116 percent (Table 7). This increment was due primarily to increase in skin blood flow, which increased by 224 percent, and, to a

* Measurements were made in conjunction with Mr. Martin Berdahl, thermodynamicist, Space Instruments Section of the Jet Propulsion Laboratory, California Institute of Technology, Pasadena.

lesser extent, muscle blood flow, which increased by 35 percent. Concomitant increases in heart rate, respiration rate, and skin and incubator temperature were observed. No significant changes were observed in rectal temperature (Table 7). In the second study, the skin temperature was kept constant at 36.5 °C before and during phototherapy by adjustment of incubator temperature. Significant increases were observed in total and skin blood flow, with mean increases of 14 and 52 percent, respectively (Table 8). Muscle blood flow, respiration, and heart rates remain unchanged (Table 8).

These findings suggest that increases in surface temperature during phototherapy and the direct effect of photoirradiation resulted in augmentation of total blood flow. Temperature change appears to affect both skin and muscle blood flow while phototherapy without change in skin temperature caused an increase in skin blood flow.

This effect of phototherapy on peripheral circulation is important for several reasons. In icteric infants exposed to phototherapy, the presence of icterus in shielded areas of the skin suggests that photooxidation occurs in the skin, and augmentation of blood flow to the skin may therefore increase the efficiency of phototherapy. How this shunting of blood to a wide skin area affects the circulatory system and cardiac output needs to be studied. Increase in peripheral blood flow may help in heat dissipation and increase evaporative losses from the skin.

TABLE 8 Changes in Blood Flow and Temperature, and Rates of Respiration and Heartbeat with Phototherapy (Second Study)

	Prephototherapy ($\overline{m} \pm 1$ SD)	Phototherapy ($\overline{m} \pm 1$ SD)	"t" Test
Blood flow (ml/100 ml tissue/min)			
Total	14.30 ± 2.45	19.48 ± 2.90	$p < 0.01$
Muscle	5.84 ± 1.40	6.73 ± 2.11	Not significant
Skin	8.46 ± 1.90	12.74 ± 2.97	$p < 0.01$
Temperature (°C)			
Skin	36.5	36.5	
Rectal	37.0 ± 0.4	36.20 ± 0.8	$p < 0.02$
Incubator	35.6 ± 1.8	34.0 ± 1.0	$p < 0.02$
Respiration (rate/min)	48.0 ± 7.0	47.0 ± 7.0	Not significant
Heartbeat (rate/min)	139.0 ± 4.0	141.0 ± 4.0	Not significant

SOURCE: Data from Wu *et al.*[21]

NOTE: The prephototherapy control groups of the first study (Table 7) and the second study exhibited greater differences in blood flow associated with the differences in skin, rectal, and incubator temperatures than did the postphototherapy study groups.

Insensible Water Loss

A series of studies on insensible water loss were done on 21 well preterm infants (mean birth weight, 1670 g). Each infant was studied twice, once before and once during phototherapy. Each study consisted of observations made during four consecutive half-hour periods. Study periods were initiated 30 min–1 h after feeding, with the infant lying naked, in a quiet state, in an incubator. Heart rate, respiration rate, and skin, rectal, and incubator temperature were recorded. Changes in body weight were measured by a Potter's Electronic Scale. Since weight of CO_2 excreted and O_2 consumed accounts for only a small proportion (10%) of IWL, they were not taken into account in the results. IWL was found to be significantly increased from a mean of 0.7 ± 0.24 (SD) ml/kg/h before phototherapy to a mean of 2.14 ± 0.40 (SD) ml/kg/h during phototherapy ($p<0.01$). Concomitant increases, similar to those obtained in the preceding blood-flow studies, were observed in heart rate, respiration rate, and skin and incubator temperature.

This increase in IWL may be due to radiant heat, from the phototherapy lamps, on the skin. In recent observations made by us,* additional far-infrared energy was present inside the incubator when the lamps were actually operating for 30 min–1 h, but was not present the instant after the lamps were turned on. The rise in skin temperature may account for vasodilatation. This, coupled with increased respiratory rate, would increase IWL. Since the vaporization of 1 g of water accounts for the loss of about 0.58 calorie of heat from the infant, IWL accounts for the dissipation of about one fourth of the heat of metabolism under basal circumstance. Phototherapy alters the environment both by photoenergy and by radiant heat. Under these circumstances, although metabolic rate may be expected to increase, the rise may not be proportional; e.g., a threefold rise in IWL during phototherapy may not represent a threefold increase in metabolic rate. In addition, because these observations on IWL were made in preterm infants, various factors—including differences in metabolic response to thermal stress due to immaturity, thickness, and water content of skin, and increased respiratory rate [2]—may also affect our results. In addition, the possibility exists that infrared energy from the lamps may be a factor in vaporization of water; however, it seems reasonable to postulate that a caloric drain imposed by increased IWL would occur during phototherapy.

* Measurements were made in conjunction with Mr. Martin Berdahl, thermodynamicist, Space Instruments Section of the Jet Propulsion Laboratory, California Institute of Technology, Pasadena.

Balance Studies

The passage of loose stools by the infant during phototherapy has been frequently noted. It seems that this could interfere with absorption of nutrients. To examine the possibility, balance studies have been performed on infants while they were receiving phototherapy; the results were compared with those obtained after phototherapy. The methods used were similar to those published by Wu *et al.*[20] Table 9 shows the results obtained from one infant. The net balance of water, nitrogen, sodium, and potassium was found to be less during phototherapy than during the control period. During the phototherapy period, the infant did not gain weight, and his measured water balance was 85.3 ml. Assuming that his IWL was about 2.1 ml/kg/h, his entire water balance was lost through IWL. The balance data from the period when he was off phototherapy indicate a net gain in weight of 25 g. This increment is compatible both with increase in body water and with increase of intracellular substance, since retention of potassium in relation to retention of nitrogen is adequate. Another interesting fact is the negative balance of sodium obtained during both balances. The negative balance is compatible with the contraction in body sodium content in infants during the first few days of life.

We were able to conduct a 2-year follow-up on 57 of the 120 infants studied. Weight, length, and head circumference were recorded as percentile of expected growth for chronologic age on the Boston-Anthropometric curve for weight and length and on Nellhaus curves for head circumference. The results are shown in Table 10. At 2 yr, there were no significant differences in measurements between the continuous or intermittently treated and the control infants.

TABLE 9 Balance Studies of One Infant (kg/24 h)

	Phototherapy Period (24 h) [a]				Control Period (24 h) [b]			
		Output				Output		
	Intake	Urine	Stool	Balance	Intake	Urine	Stool	Balance
H_2O (ml)	156.5	74.1	19.2	85.3	189.1	65.8	7.4	115.9
N (g)	0.59	0.12	0.12	0.35	0.71	0.10	0.06	0.54
Na (m*M*)	2.39	4.37	0.29	−2.27	2.89	2.96	0.41	−0.21
K (m*M*)	3.70	1.7	1.05	0.94	4.48	0.99	0.43	3.06

[a] Initial weight (wt_i) = 1520; final weight (wt_f) = 1520.
[b] Wt_i = 1525; wt_f = 1550.

TABLE 10 Phototherapy Follow-up, 1970–1971 Study, at 2 Years of Age

	Phototherapy Group					
	Continuous (A)		Intermittent (B)		Control (C)	
Parameter [a]	No.	%	No.	%	No.	%
Weight < 10%	6	32	2	11	9	47
Body Length < 10%	9	47	8	44	7	37
Head circumference < 2%	2	10	0	—	2	10
Total No. Retested	19		18		20	

[a] Parameters are those for normal growth for this age on the Boston-Anthropometric curve (for weight and body length) and Nellhaus curve (for head circumference).

The data from these studies suggest the need for further observation of the biological effects of photoirradiation on infants. Appropriate increase in fluid and caloric intake may compensate for the increased insensible water loss (IWL) and caloric drain. The follow-up results appear to be reassuring.

Acknowledgments

Other co-investigators involved with various parts of the studies reported here were Joan E. Hodgman, M.D., Rosie Lim, M.D., Mary Kokosky, M.D., Annabel Teberg, M.D., Woon Wong, M.D., and Norman Levan, M.D.

REFERENCES

1. Echave Llanos, J. M., M. D. Aloisso, M. Souto, R. Balduzzi, and J. M. Surur. Circadian variations of DNA synthesis, mitotic activity, and cell size of hepatocyte population in young immature male mouse growing liver. Virchows Arch. 8:309–317, 1971.
2. Fanaroff, A. A., M. Wald, H. S. Gruber, and M. H. Klaus. Insensible water loss in low birth weight infants. Pediatrics 50:236–245, 1972.
3. Hollwich, F. Experimentelle Untersuchungen über die Beziehungen des energetischen Anteiles der Sehbahn zu der Regeneration des Blutes. Münch. Med. Wochenschr. 95:212–214, 1953.
4. Hyman, C., T. Greeson, M. Clem, and D. Winsor. Capacitance–plethysmograph method for separating blood flow in muscle and skin in the human forearm. Am. Heart J. 68:508–514, 1964.
5. Jones, M. F., and A. Hollaender. The effect of long ultraviolet and near

visible radiation on the eggs of the nematodes, *Enterobius vermicularis* and *Ascaris lumbricoides*. J. Parasitol. 28 (Dec. Suppl.): 17–18, 1942. (A)

6. Lewis, T. The Blood Vessels of the Human Skin and their Responses, p. 117. London: Shaw, 1927.
7. Licht, S. H., Ed. Therapeutic Electricity and Ultraviolet Radiation, p. 262. Baltimore: Waverly Press, 1959.
8. Lucey, J. F. Phototherapy of jaundice 1969. Birth Defects 6:63–70, 1970.
9. Malyuk, V. I., and V. M. Fomicheva. The diurnal dynamics of DNA synthesis in cells of the thoracic duct wall. Autoradiographic study. Antiologica 8:1–6, 1971.
10. Morgan, W. W., and S. Mizell. Diurnal fluctuation in DNA content and DNA synthesis in the dorsal epidermis of *Rana pipiens*. Comp. Biochem. Physiol. 38:591–602, 1971.
11. Morris, T. R. The effect of light intensity on growing and laying pullets. World Poult. Sci. J. 23:246–252, 1967.
12. Nir, I., N. Hirschmann, and F. G. Sulman. Diurnal rhythms of pineal nucleic acids and protein. Neuroendocrinology 7:271–277, 1971.
13. Ott, J. N. Effects of wavelengths of light on physiological functions of plants and animals. Illum. Eng. 60:254–261, 1965.
14. Plexiglass Design and Fabric Data, p. 19105. Bulletin PL53G. Philadelphia: Rohm and Haas Co., June 1971.
15. Scholz, K., and C. Lips. Zur Frage des Lichteinflusses auf die Mast-und Schlachtleistung von Schweinen. Tierzucht 18:639–640, 1964.
16. Squibb, R. L. Effect of lighting regimen on simultaneous diurnal rhythms of nucleic and free amino acids in the liver, heart, intestine and pancreas of the chick. Poult. Sci. 50:486–491, 1971.
17. Tamimie, H. S. Influence of different light regimens on the growth and sexual maturity of chickens. Growth 31:183–189, 1967.
18. Tamimie, H. S. Light exposure of incubating eggs and its influence on the growth of chicks. I. Brooding chicks under different light regimens. Comp. Biochem. Physiol. 21:59–63, 1967.
19. Tamimie, H. S., and M. W. Fox. Effect of continuous and intermittent light exposure on the embryonic development of chicken eggs. Comp. Biochem. Physiol. 20:793–799, 1967.
20. Wu, P. Y. K., W. Oh, A. Lubetkin, and J. Metcoff. "Late edema" in low birth weight infants. Pediatrics 41:67–76, 1968.
21. Wu, P. Y. K., W. H. Wong, J. E. Hodgman, and N. Levan. Changes in blood flow in the skin and muscle with phototherapy. Pediatr. Res. 8:257–262, 1974.
22. Wu, P. Y. K., T. Yoshida, J. E. Hodgman, and B. Siassi. Cellular growth changes in newborn rats exposed to phototherapy. Pediatr. Res. 6:431/171, 1972. (A)
23. Wurtman, R. J. The pineal and endocrine function. Hosp. Pract. 4:32–37, 1969.
24. Yasunaga, S., and E. H. Kean. The effect of Plexiglas incubators on phototherapy. J. Pediatr. 81:89–90, 1972.

RICHARD J. WURTMAN

Effects of Light on Man

Light and Biological Rhythms

The amount of time that all living things are exposed to light varies with two cycles: a 24-hour, light–dark cycle of day and night and an annual cycle of changing day length, absent only at the equator. These light cycles correspond to many rhythmic changes in mammalian biological functions: Motor activity, sleep, food and water consumption, body temperature, and the rates at which many glands secrete their hormones—all these vary with rhythms whose periods approximate 24 h (Table 1). Thus, the concentration of cortisol in the blood of human subjects has a characteristic 24-hour rhythm; it is maximal in the morning hours and attains its nadir in the evening. When people reverse their activity cycles (for example, by working during the hours of darkness and sleeping during daylight), their plasma cortisol rhythms require 5–10 days to adapt to the new environmental conditions.[7]

Annual rhythms in sexual activity, hibernation, and migratory behavior are also widespread among animal species. The physiological significance of such rhythms probably derives from their ability to synchronize the activities of multiple members of a species to each other and to enable the animals to "anticipate" annual cycles of changing environmental conditions. For example, sheep ovulate and are fertilized in the

TABLE 1 Some Rhythmic Functions in Man

Rhythmic Function	Usual Time of Peak Level or Activity
Sleep	1–4 a.m.
Eosinophils in blood	1–3 a.m.
ACTH in plasma	2–5 a.m.
Cortisol in plasma	6–9 a.m.
Magnesium and calcium in urine	9–11 a.m.
17-Hydroxycorticosteroids in urine	10–12 a.m.
Sodium and potassium in urine	1–3 p.m.
Wakefulness	1–4 p.m.
Urine volume	3–6 p.m.
Catecholamine metabolites in urine	4–7 p.m.
Body temperature	4–6 p.m.
Skin reaction to subcutaneously injected histamine	7–11 p.m.
Phosphates in urine	10–12 p.m.

fall, thus anticipating the spring by many months, when food will be available to the mother for nursing the newborn. For humans, the adaptive pressures of cyclic changes in the environment appear to be of less significance. Psychosocial factors probably are of greater importance than light cycles in generating or synchronizing biological rhythms. The biological utility to humans of having a sleep–wakefulness rhythm, or of other rhythms that follow from it, remains to be identified.

Cycles in environmental lighting may interact with biological rhythms in several ways. The light cycle may *induce* the rhythm; in this event, placing a mammal in an environment of continuous light or darkness should rapidly abolish the rhythm. Thus, the content of norepinephrine in the rat pineal varies each day with a characteristic rhythm, but the rhythm disappears in the absence of day–night light cycles.[21] (The neuroanatomic and physiological mechanisms by which environmental lighting affects pineal metabolism are described below.) Another cyclic environmental input—dietary protein—has also been shown to generate a daily rhythm. Amino acids consumed as protein travel to the liver via the portal circulation after each meal and cause the protein-synthesizing units (polysomes) to become aggregated. This accelerates the synthesis of a hepatic enzyme, tyrosine transaminase.[8, 22]

Rather than *inducing* the rhythm, the light cycle might simply *entrain* it, causing all animals in the same species to exhibit maxima and minima at about the same times of day or night. The factor that generates the rhythmicity *per se* could be a different cyclic environmental input (such as dietary protein) or an intrinsic oscillator (perhaps that metaphysical monstrosity, the "biological clock"). In either case, placing the mammal in an environment of continuous light or darkness should not extinguish the rhythm. If the rhythmic chemical or physical process can be sampled repeatedly in the same animal, it is possible to show that in the absence of a cyclic lighting input the rhythms in different animals become dissociated from one another. Presumably this dissociation occurs because the rhythm "free-runs" or becomes "circadian";[1, 10, 14] that is, its precise period changes from exactly 24 h to something that is more or less characteristic for each animal. If the rhythm does free-run, this is good evidence that it is not generated by a cyclic environmental input exhibiting 24-hour periodicity (such as light, ambient temperature, or humidity). It could, of course, be generated by other cyclic environmental inputs (such as food and water consumption) that also free-run in the absence of light; or it could result from intrinsic oscillators. In any case, only a few rhythms are amenable to this sort of experimental analysis in mammals, since only rhythms in behavior, body temperature, and plasma and urinary concentrations can conveniently be studied by repeatedly sampling the same subject.

Relatively little information is available concerning the action spectra or intensities required for light to generate or entrain daily rhythms in mammals; it is known that light is the dominant environmental input affecting rhythms and that light exerts its effects indirectly via retinal photoreceptors. The action spectrum for the entrainment of the body temperature rhythm in rats[12] is similar to that required for the inhibition of the rat pineal[4] and to the absorption spectrum of rhodopsin.[17] (See Figure 1.)

Light and the Mammalian Pineal Organ

Of all the indirect effects of light on mammalian processes, the photic control of hormone synthesis in the pineal organ is, next to vision, the best characterized. The great current interest in the pineal organ was probably initiated by Lerner's discovery of its hormone, melatonin, in 1959. Experiments performed subsequently have shown that nervous impulses reaching the pineal via its sympathetic nerves control the rate at which this organ synthesizes melatonin.[20] These impulses vary inversely with the amount of visible light impinging on the retinas.[16] They are carried through the brain, spinal cord, and sympathetic nervous system by a circuitous route that differs from the pathway responsible for vision (Figure 2).

If rats are maintained for several days under conditions of continuous

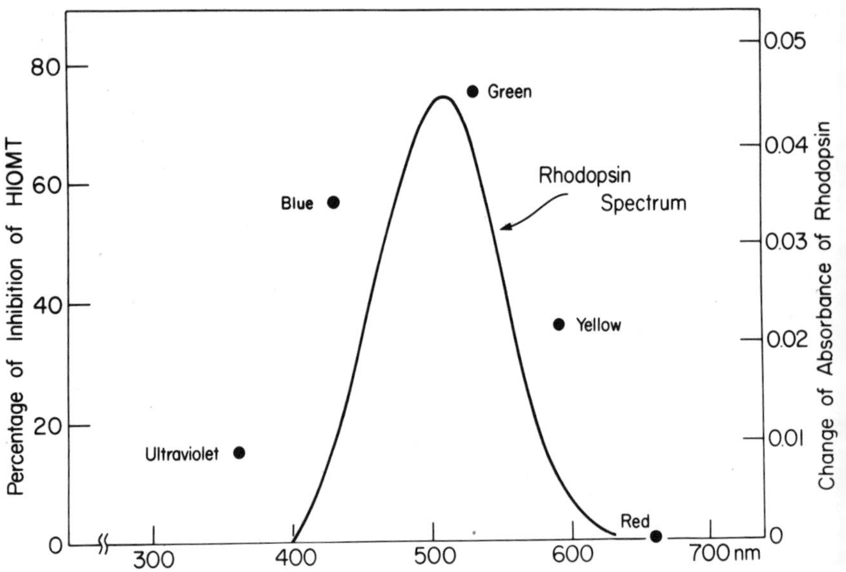

FIGURE 1 Inhibition of the pineal enzyme hydroxyindole-*O*-methyl transferase (HIOMT) by light of various colors. Groups of rats were exposed to five narrow-spectrum light sources (ultraviolet, blue, green, yellow, and red) for 96 h each. These sources were all at the same level of radiant energy (65 $\mu W/cm^2$). The percentage of inhibition of the melatonin-synthesizing enzyme is co-plotted with the absorption spectrum of rhodopsin, the visual pigment present in the rat retina. (From Cardinali *et al.*[4])

illumination, the activities of the pineal enzymes involved in melatonin biosynthesis decrease manyfold.[19] This effect is absent in animals whose eyes have been removed or in which the nerves to the pineal have been cut. The decrease in pineal enzyme activity appears to be an exaggeration of the "normal" response of the pineal to natural light cycles; melatonin synthesis is also slowest at the end of the daily light period among animals kept in a cyclically lighted environment.[2] Although the precise role of melatonin (the main pineal hormone thus far characterized) in the physiology of the intact mammal has not yet been ascertained, it is well established that its administration affects the secretion by various endocrine organs, probably by acting on neuroendocrine control centers in the brain.[20] It also induces sleep, modifies the electroencephalogram, and raises the levels of the neurotransmitter serotonin in the brain. Melatonin administration blocks the cyclic release of the luteinizing hormone—the hormone responsible for ovulation—from the anterior pituitary gland. Immature rats kept under continuous illumination became sex-

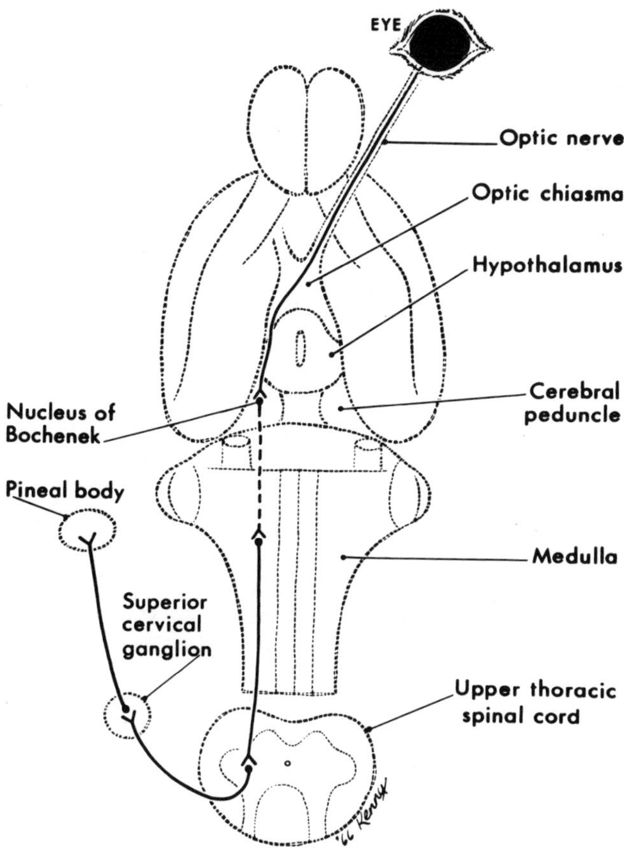

FIGURE 2 Representation of neural pathways by which light indirectly controls the synthesis of the pineal hormone melatonin. Light stimuli reach the pineal by a circuitous route ultimately involving the sympathetic nervous system. Photoreceptors in the eye respond to environmental lighting by generating nerve impulses that are transmitted along the optic nerve. Most of these impulses travel to brain centers that are associated with vision. A small fraction diverge from the main visual pathway and, instead, travel along a nerve bundle (the inferior accessory optic tract) that leads to the central hypothalamic neurons involved in the regulation of the sympathetic nervous system. From this point, the pathway descends via the spinal cord to the preganglionic neurons supplying the superior cervical ganglia; the postganglionic neurons then ascend to the pineal where they act by liberating the neurotransmitter norepinephrine. Norepinephrine enhances the activity of several pineal enzymes involved in the synthesis of melatonin. (From Wurtman *et al.*[20])

ually mature at an earlier age than animals kept under a 24-hour, light–dark cycle; [18] this effect may have been mediated by the photic inhibition of melatonin secretion.

In summary, although the mammalian pineal is not directly responsive to light, its secretory activity is controlled by light. The secretion of melatonin by the pineal may serve to synchronize the lighting environment with intrinsic biological processes that are not primarily dependent on light. In certain lower vertebrates, the pineal is directly responsive to environmental lighting,[6, 15] serving as a photoreceptive "third eye" that sends messages about the state of environmental lighting to the brain. In the mammalian pineal organ, all such traces of direct photoreceptive function appear to be lost. The retinal photoreceptor that mediates the control of the mammalian pineal by light has not yet been identified. Recent studies suggest, however, that this photoreceptor utilizes rhodopsin and may thus be a rod cell.[4] Figure 1 illustrates the similarity between the action spectrum for the photic inhibition of pineal HIOMT (hydroxyindole-*O*-methyl transferase), an enzyme required for melatonin biosynthesis, and the absorption spectrum for rhodopsin. The intensity of white light required to cause a 50-percent suppression of pineal biosynthetic activity in the intact rat is about 0.5 $\mu W/cm^2$ (K. Minneman, H. Lynch, M. Hsuan, and R. J. Wurtman, *Life Sciences,* in press).

Light and Mammalian Gonadal Function

Environmental lighting has been shown to influence the maturation and subsequent cyclic activity of the gonads in all mammalian and avian species thus far examined.[18] The particular responses of each species to light seem to depend on whether the species is monoestrous or polyestrous—that is, whether it normally ovulates once a year (in the spring or fall) or at regular intervals throughout the year. Examples of the latter are laboratory rats (every 4–5 days); guinea pigs (every 12–14 days); and humans (every 29 days). The gonadal responses of each species to light also seem to depend on whether its members are physically active during the daylight hours or during the nighttime. Thus, if weanling rats (a nocturnal, polyestrous species) are kept from birth under continuous illumination, they mature at a younger age than control animals kept under cyclic illumination, but then they fail to ovulate cyclically, exhibiting instead a state of "persistent estrus." [18] Blindness in humans (a diurnally active, polyestrous species) is also associated with early gonadal maturation.[23] (See Table 2.) The gonads of most birds and of most diurnally active, monoestrous mammals mature in the springtime, in response to the gradual increase in day length. Ovulation can be accelerated in these animals by exposing them to arti-

TABLE 2 Effect of Blindness on Age of Menarche in Humans [a]

Group [b]		Number	Mean Age (mo)	SD	SE
IA	Premature, blind [c]	85	143.0	14.5	1.6 [d]
IB	Premature, blind	107	144.0	14.3	1.4 [d]
II	Premature, nonblind	98	150.8	16.1	1.6
III	Term, blind [e]	68 [f]	146.0	14.6	1.9 [g]
IV	Term, nonblind	235	150.5	10.2	0.7

[a] Derived from Zacharias and Wurtman.[23]
[b] Girls in Group IA had no light perception; those in Group IB had some.
[c] Prematurely born girls.
[d] Differs from Group II, $p < 0.01$.
[e] Girls born at full term.
[f] The nine subjects in this group without light perception were not included in the study.
[g] Differs from Group IV, $p < 0.01$.

ficial "long days." The annual period of gonadal activity in domestic sheep (a diurnally active, monoestrous species) occurs in the fall, in response to decreasing day length. The mechanisms that cause some species to be monoestrous and others polyestrous, or that cause some animals to sleep by day and others by night, are entirely unknown, as are those that cause wide variation in the gonadal responses of various species to light.

In birds, photoreceptors capable of mediating gonadal responses apparently exist in the brain as well as in the eyes; hence, light reaching the brain of the duck via quartz rods placed in the eye sockets can be used to accelerate gonadal enlargement.[3] In adult mammals, however, only the retinas appear to contain the photoreceptor cells necessary for stimulating gonadal responses (or any other neuroendocrine effects, for that matter). In support of this conclusion, removal of the eyes completely blocks the ability of experimental illumination to accelerate maturation or to interfere with the mechanisms responsible for causing ovulation.[18] The neural and neuroendocrine pathways connecting the retinas and the gonads are poorly defined. One such pathway probably involves the pineal organ and melatonin;[20] another may utilize cells in the hypothalamus, which, by secreting "releasing factors," control the secretion of gonadotropin hormones from the anterior pituitary. The action spectra for the effects of light on mammalian gonads have not been identified.

Light and Vitamin D

Vitamin D_3, or cholecalciferol, is formed in the skin and subcutaneous tissue when ultraviolet light is absorbed by its provitamin, 7-dehydrotachysterol; it can also be obtained by eating fish. The precise action spectrum for the activation of the provitamin *in vivo* is not known; it may include both midultraviolet (290–320 nm) and long-wave ultraviolet (320–400 nm) irradiations. A related biologically active compound, vitamin D_2, can be obtained by consuming milk and other foods fortified with irradiated ergosterol (ergocalciferol); however, it remains to be demonstrated that this exogenous source is as biologically effective as the vitamin D formed in the skin. In a population of Caucasian adults from St. Louis, Missouri, 71–91 percent of the total vitamin D activity in the blood was observed to be associated with vitamin D_3 and its derivatives;[9] hence, sunlight remains vastly more important than food as a source of vitamin D.

Recent studies by DeLuca and others have shown that vitamin D compounds are further transformed by the liver and kidneys to more active metabolites that are hydroxylated at the 1 and 25 positions; these metabolites act on the intestinal mucosa to facilitate calcium absorption, and on bone to facilitate calcium exchange.[5] Loomis has suggested that the term *vitamin D* is a misnomer; the active compound is normally synthesized endogenously and thus is much more a hormone than a vitamin.[11] Like the hormone thyroxine, which cannot be synthesized in the absence of the dietary constituent iodine, the hormone vitamin D cannot be formed in the absence of the environmental input light. Just as one could substitute the consumption of irradiated milk for exposing oneself to sunlight, a person could replace his need for dietary iodine by consuming bovine thyroids. This does not mean that thyroxine should be considered a vitamin.

It has been recognized for some years that children chronically exposed to inadequate amounts of sunlight may develop rickets, a deforming disease characterized by undermineralization of the bones. This disease can be cured by irradiating the skin with ultraviolet light or by feeding afflicted children 200–400 IU of vitamin D daily.[11] Recent studies in Boston showed that apparently normal, elderly males deprived of ultraviolet light for 3 months (by remaining indoors during the winter in environments illuminated by standard incandescent or fluorescent sources) developed an impairment in the ability of their intestinal mucosa to absorb calcium. Concurrent exposure of similar males for 8 h/d to a lighting environment designed to simulate the solar spectrum in the visible and near-ultraviolet ranges blocked the 40-percent fall in calcium absorption observed in the control subjects.[13] (See Figure 3.) The amount of ultraviolet light impinging on these subjects was equivalent to the amount that they might be expected to receive during a 15-minute lunch-time walk in the summer. It seems possible that the appropriate design

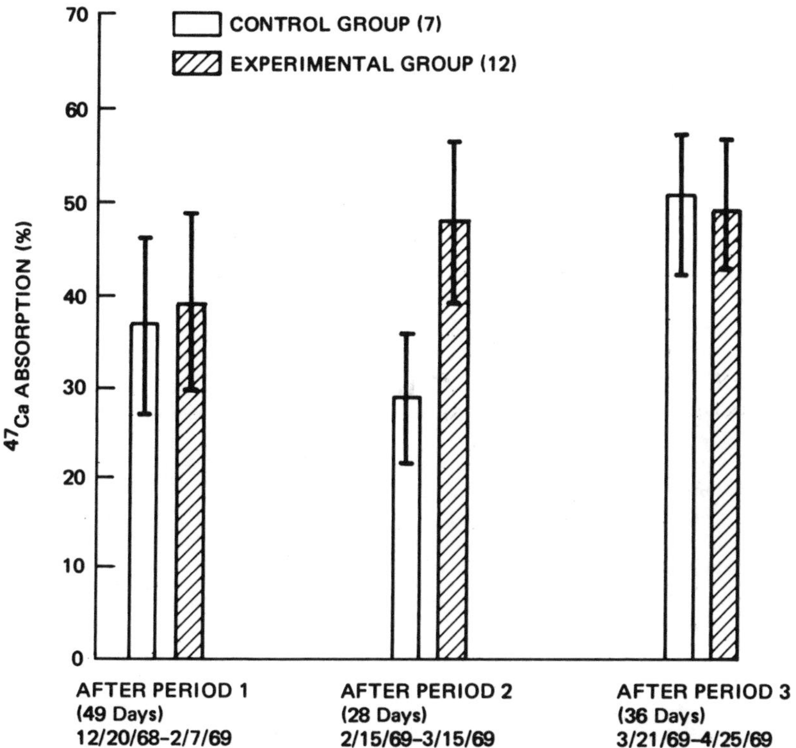

FIGURE 3 Stimulation of calcium absorption in elderly human subjects by artificial lighting. From December 20, 1968, to April 25, 1969, 18 healthy males between 57 and 80 years of age were asked to stay indoors and away from open windows during daylight. Twelve subjects were considered the experimental group and six were considered the controls. During Period 1, all subjects were exposed to regular fluorescent lighting; at the end of this period the ability of each subject to absorb calcium was estimated by measuring the percentage of ^{47}Ca passed in feces within 6 days of ingestion. During Period 2, the 12 experimental subjects were exposed to an artificial sunlight illuminant (Vita-Lite) while the 7 controls remained under regular fluorescent luminaires that lacked significant ultraviolet emissions. At the end of this period, ^{47}Ca absorption was again measured. In Period 3, all subjects were again exposed to the conditions of artificial light used during Period 1. Differences between experimental and control groups after Period 2 were significant ($p < 0.01$). (From Neer *et al.*[13])

of artificial lighting environments could provide a powerful public health measure for the prophylaxis of undermineralization of the skeleton.

REFERENCES

1. Aschoff, J., Ed. Circadian Clocks. Amsterdam: North Holland Publishing Co., 1965. 479 pp.
2. Axelrod, J., R. J. Wurtman, and S. H. Snyder. Control of hydroxyindole *O*-methyltransferase activity in the rat pineal gland by environmental lighting. J. Biol. Chem. 240:949–954, 1965.
3. Benoit, J., and I. Assenmacher. The control by visible radiations of the gonadotropic activity of the duck hypophysis. Recent Prog. Hormone Res. 15:143–164, 1959.
4. Cardinali, D. P., F. Larin, and R. J. Wurtman. Control of the rat pineal gland by light spectra (melatonin hydroxyindole-*O*-methyl transferase). Proc. Natl. Acad. Sci. (USA) 69:2003–2005, 1972.
5. DeLuca, H. F. Role of kidney tissue in metabolism of vitamin D. N. Engl. J. Med. 284:554, 1971.
6. Dodt, E., and E. Heerd. Mode of action of pineal nerve fibers in frogs. J. Neurophysiol. 25:405–429, 1962.
7. Eisenstein, A. M., Ed. The Adrenal Cortex. Boston: Little, Brown and Co., 1967. 685 pp.
8. Fishman, B., R. J. Wurtman, and H. N. Munro. Daily rhythms in hepatic polysome profiles and tyrosine transaminase activity: Role of dietary protein. Proc. Natl. Acad. Sci. (USA) 64:677–682, 1969.
9. Haddad, J. G., Jr., and T. J. Hahn. Natural and synthetic sources of circulating 25-hydroxyvitamin D in man. Nature 244:515–517, 1973.
10. Halberg, F. Circadian (about twenty-four-hour) rhythms in experimental medicine. Proc. R. Soc. Med. 56:253–260, 1963.
11. Loomis, W. F. Rickets. Sci. Am. 223:76–91, 1970.
12. McGuire, R. A., W. M. Rand, and R. J. Wurtman. Entrainment of the body temperature rhythm in rats: Effect of color and intensity of environmental light. Science 181:956–957, 1973.
13. Neer, R. M., T. R. A. Davis, A. Walcott, S. Koski, P. Schepis, I. Taylor, L. Thorington, and R. J. Wurtman. Stimulation by artificial lighting of calcium absorption in elderly human subjects. Nature 229:255–257, 1971.
14. Pittendrigh, C. S., and S. D. Skopik. Circadian systems, V. The driving oscillation and the temporal sequence of development. Proc. Natl. Acad. Sci. (USA) 65:500–507, 1970.
15. Rosner, J. M., G. D. Pérez Bedéz, and D. P. Cardinali. Direct effect of light on duck pineal explants. Life Sci. (Part II) 10:1065–1069, 1971.
16. Taylor, A. N., and R. W. Wilson. Electrophysiological evidence for the action of light on the pineal gland in the rat. Experientia 26:267–269, 1970.
17. Wald, G. The receptors of human color vision. Science 145:1007–1016, 1964.
18. Wurtman, R. J. Effects of light and visual stimuli on endocrine function, pp. 19–59. In L. Martini and W. F. Ganong, Eds. Neuroendocrinology. Vol. 2. New York: Academic Press, Inc., 1967.
19. Wurtman, R. J., J. Axelrod, and J. E. Fischer. Melatonin synthesis in the

pineal gland: Effect of light mediated by the sympathetic nervous system. Science 143:1328–1330, 1964.

20. Wurtman, R. J., J. Axelrod, and D. E. Kelly. The Pineal. New York: Academic Press, Inc., 1968. 199 pp.
21. Wurtman, R. J., J. Axelrod, G. Sedvall, and R. Y. Moore. Photic and neural control of the 24-hour epinephrine rhythm in the rat pineal gland. J. Pharmacol. Exp. Ther. 157:487–492, 1967.
22. Wurtman, R. J., W. J. Shoemaker, and F. Larin. Mechanism of the daily rhythm in hepatic tyrosine transaminase activity: Role of dietary tryptophan. Proc. Natl. Acad. Sci. (USA) 59:800–807, 1968.
23. Zacharias, L., and R. J. Wurtman. Blindness and menarche. Obstet. Gynecol. 33:603–608, 1969.

J. W. HASTINGS

Circadian Rhythms

Effect of Light on Circadian Rhythms

Since the introduction of jet travel, most of us have become more aware of our internal rhythms, or at least of the fact that shifting the phase of the daily "synchronization" can cause discomfort, if not actual physiological disruptions. Although human rhythms have been known for a long time,[1, 11, 17] it is only recently that their semiautonomy has been appreciated along with their truly important interaction with various functional systems.[3–5, 12, 20, 24]

By semiautonomy we mean that there exists an internal clocklike mechanism and that these rhythmic changes are not simply a direct response to the environmental periodicities associated with the rotation of the earth, to which all life on this planet is subjected and wherein it evolved. The environmental periodicities are nevertheless important in driving and entraining our rhythms, which indicates that the rhythmic system is not completely autonomous. So, in considering any kind of phototherapy, it is appropriate to inquire what effect the exposure to light might be expected to have upon the circadian semiautonomous daily rhythms. For example, should the light regime be designed to simulate a normal night and day? Could a continuous exposure to a bright light, which is known to inhibit rhythmic phenomena in animals, have an adverse effect on rhythmicity and the attendant physiological phenomena? There are, to be sure, very few experiments that impinge directly on these questions, so the best one can do is to give educated guesses. In my judgment, possible adverse effects on physiological rhythms should not be used as a strong argument against phototherapy. On the time scale of physiological rhythms, the duration of the treatment is short (2–4 days), and it therefore seems unlikely that serious or permanent injury to the rhythmic system would occur. Nevertheless, I consider it essential that experimental phototherapy include protocols addressed to questions concerning circadian rhythmicity.

Biology of Circadian Rhythms

Much of the important evidence concerning the existence and properties of our "biological clock" comes from studies with relatively simple systems, but most of the key properties have been demonstrated also in human subjects, or in mammals, or in both. These key properties include first the fact that rhythmicity continues under constant laboratory conditions with a period that is close to, but usually is not exactly, 24 h—thus, circadian, or about 1 day.

Second, rhythms can be entrained by environmental periodicities that themselves have periods close to the periodicities of the "natural" or circadian period: Cycles of light, temperature, and possibly sound or other physical and chemical factors are effective. Such a factor is referred to as a *zeitgeber*. Phase shifting represents another aspect of this phenomenon. After traveling rapidly across the ocean, your sleep–wake cycle shifts or adjusts to local time, perhaps only after some days of physiological disturbance. Similarly, circadian rhythms can be phase shifted.

Finally, a very interesting property of rhythms is that the period or frequency is almost independent of temperature. Most chemical and biological reactions are greater by a factor of 2 or 3 at a temperature 10 °C higher, but biological clocks are generally only slightly changed—usually by less than 10 percent.

To illustrate the fact that a rhythm will persist in the absence of the normal day–night cycle, I like to show the experiment of Rawson [21] (Figure 1), which recorded the running activity of a female adult *Peromyscus* for 22 days in constant darkness. The chart records of the activity are arranged in chronological order—Day 2 below Day 1, Day 3 below Day 2, and so on. The resulting pattern makes it easy to see that on each day the activity began a little earlier than it did the day before. The stages by which the periods of activity became earlier are surpris-

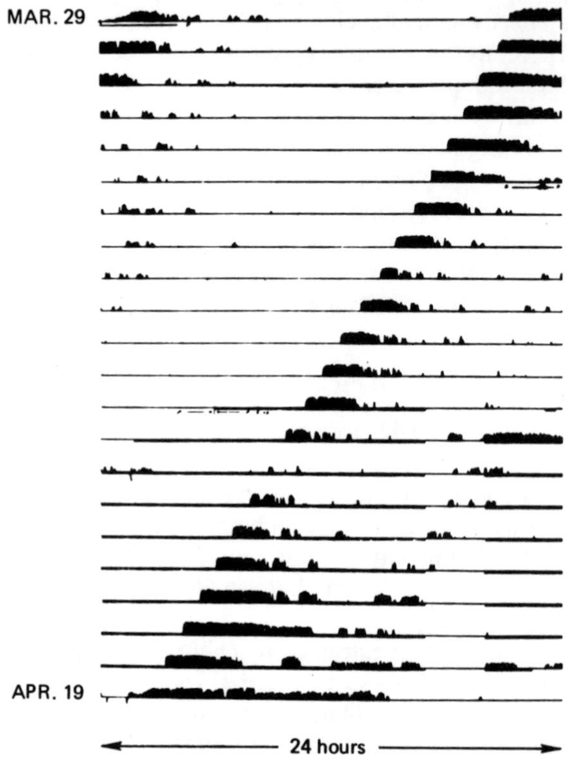

FIGURE 1 Twenty-two-day record of running activity of a female adult *Peromyscus* in constant darkness. The abscissa shows a 24-hour time span running from left to right, and the ordinate successive days from top to bottom. The ordinate of each daily record indicates the number of revolutions of running wheel per minute. The maximum rate shown is about 125 rpm. The period of rhythm is 23 h 10 min. (From Rawson.[21] Copyright 1959 by the American Association for the Advancement of Science.)

ingly regular; each day's activity began about 50 minutes earlier than the previous day's activity. The rhythm continued to occur in the absence of environmental clues, and it also had its own "natural period," which in this case was less than 24 h.

A similar experiment with a human subject is shown in Figure 2. Here the subject was entrained by "normal" 24-hour conditions for the first several days and then allowed to determine his own daily schedule without, it is believed, any references to or clues from the outside. With a

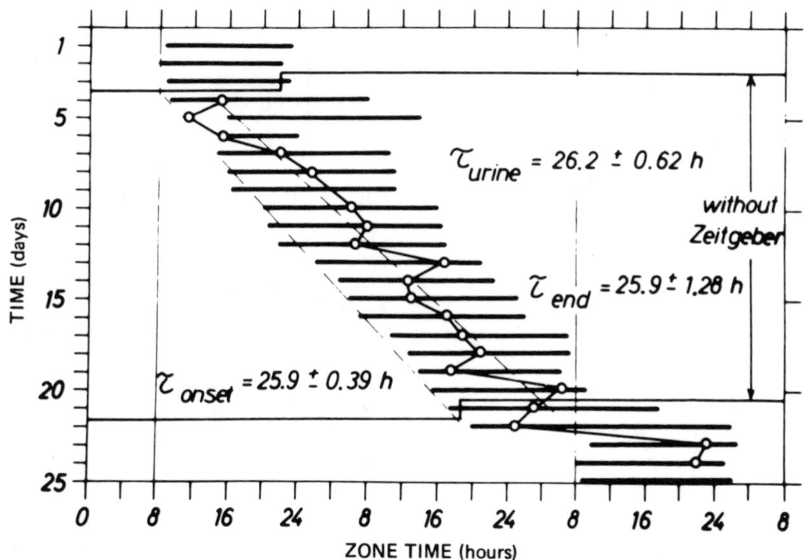

FIGURE 2 Circadian rhythm of activity and urine excretion in a human subject kept for 3 days under normal conditions, then for 18 days in isolation, and finally again under normal conditions. Black bars indicate times of being awake, the circles maxima of urine excretion, and the numbers mean values of periods for onset and end of activity and for urine maxima. (From Aschoff.[2])

natural period of about 26 h, he "lived" longer (but fewer) days; during the 20 days in isolation without zeitgeber he had scanned across the day 1½ times. At the end, he was about 12 h out of phase. When then exposed to the zeitgebers of the outside world, he made the big phase shift. This experiment shows that a person with a 26-hour natural period possesses a 24-hour rhythm when entrained by a 24-hour zeitgeber cycle, which can be interpreted as resulting from a daily reset or phase shift of 2 h. But entrainment is not necessary for phase shifting. When an organism is kept under constant conditions (Figure 3), single exposures to light, simulating dawn or dusk, can reset a biological clock with full effectiveness. The effectiveness of such a reset signal is very different, however, at different times of day.

I have already mentioned that the biological clock is only slightly affected by temperature. This so-called independence is illustrated in Figure 4, for the rhythm of luminescence of *Gonyaulax*. Here one sees an unusual result. The system is apparently *slower* at higher temperatures, but in this instance the difference is not great—only about 30 per-

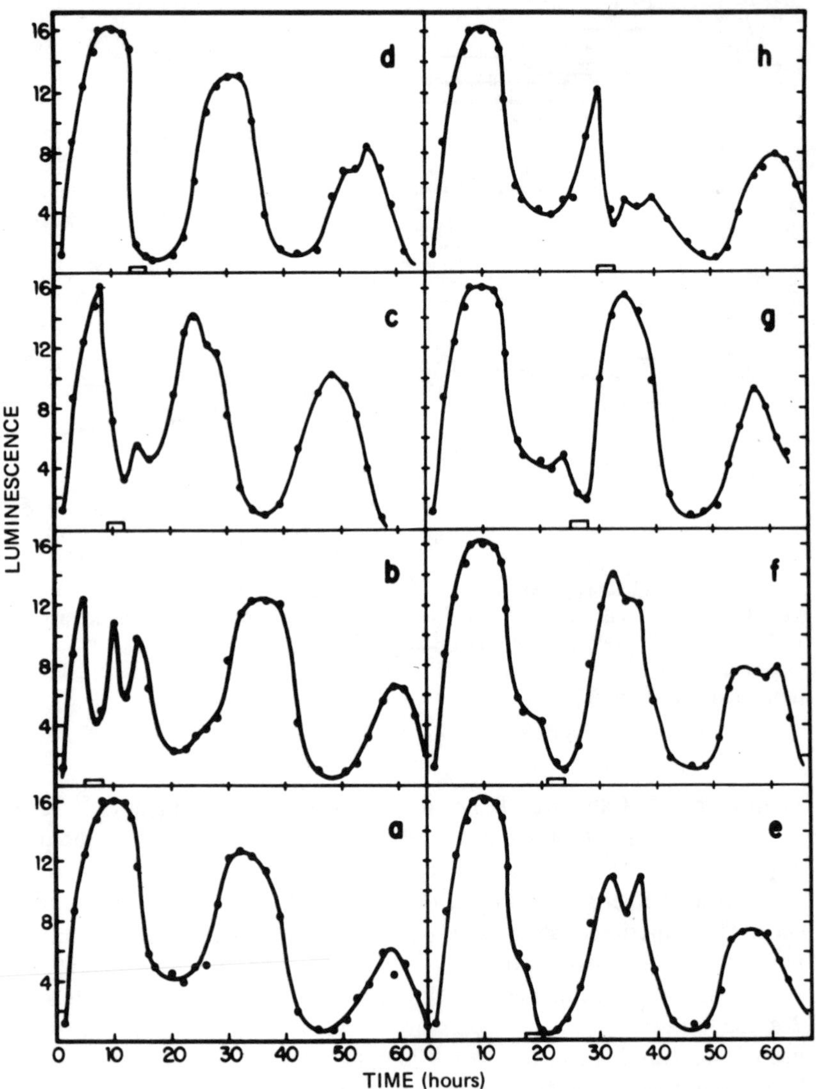

FIGURE 3 These experiments illustrate the way in which the phase of the rhythm of luminescence is shifted following an exposure of the cells to 2½-hour light pulse and the 1400 ft-c, 21 °C. Prior to the time shown on the graph, all cultures were in light:dark 12:12 conditions, and at the end of a light period the cells were placed in the dark and the control remained in the dark thereafter. The times at which light pulses were administered varied as indicated by bars on graph. Luminescence in arbitrary units. (From Hastings.[14])

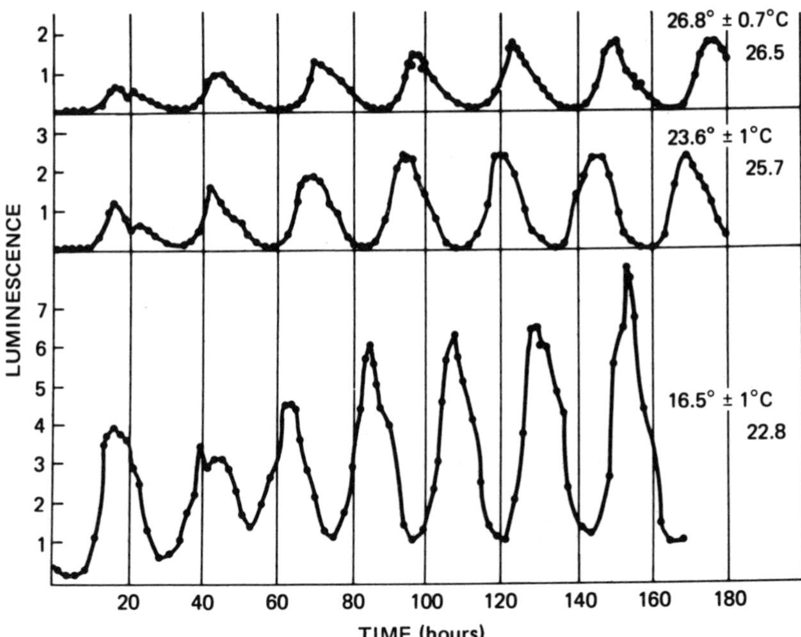

FIGURE 4 Characteristics of the persistent rhythm of luminescence in *Gonyaulax* at three different temperatures. The cells were grown in conditions of light:dark 12:12 h at 22 °C and transferred at the end of a dark period to constant light (100 ft-c) at 0 time on the graph. The luminescence capacity was measured approximately every 2 h. The average period in hours measured for each is noted on the graph below the temperature. Luminescence in arbitrary units. (From Hastings and Sweeney.[15])

cent for 10 °C. In fact, if one adopts the view that rhythms relate to a truly functional clock mechanism, this property is not a surprise; it is expected. The mechanism whereby this is achieved has not been elucidated, but it is probably appropriate to view it as temperature compensation, not temperature independence. That is, we believe that the component parts of the rhythmic mechanism are affected by temperature but that the system is assembled in such a way that the mechanism functions (so far as frequency is concerned) in a relatively temperature-independent fashion. By experimental manipulation of body temperature, it has been shown that the clock in mammals is also temperature compensated.

Continuous light has some well-known and important effects upon rhythmic systems. Most important for our consideration is the fact that circadian rhythmicity may be inhibited, or abolished, or somehow is not expressed in constant light (Figure 5). This effect may be intensity dependent; in some organisms, it occurs only at very high light intensities (Figure 6). Although I believe that the rhythmic mechanism is actually inoperative, some authors have maintained that it is only the expression of the rhythm that is abolished, and that the underlying mechanism continues.

The molecular and cellular mechanisms controlling the biological clock are not well understood. Various aspects of this problem are being studied in my laboratory. Many workers have thought in terms of some chemical "loop"—that is, a series of sequential reactions that serve to trigger in some way a series of discrete functions at various times in a recurring fashion.[13] Considerable attention has been given to the possibility that this loop somehow involves the genome (for example, RNA transcription followed by protein synthesis). Goodwin [10] and Ehret and Trucco [8] have developed this hypothesis in some detail at the theoretical level, but the experimental evidence remains spotty and insecure—particularly when one takes into account the evidence from all systems.

A second and quite different idea conceives of the clock as a biochemical network with self-sustained oscillations arising from feedback within the biochemical system.[18] In molecular terms, the network has sometimes been equated with a series of cross-inhibited (or activated) enzymes in a metabolic pathway,[19] but other ideas, especially the idea that membranes and membrane transport might be involved, have recently been put forward.[6, 9] *

Human Circadian Rhythms: Adults [7, 16, 23]

Aschoff [1] states that some 50 functions in man have been studied and shown to exhibit an autonomous circadian rhythm. These rhythmic phenomena range from those relating to basic cellular and tissue phenomena to those involving organ and organismal functions. In addition to temperature, excretory, and activity rhythms, there are circadian rhythms of cell division, heart rate, and serum content of specific substances. More elusive phenomena, such as ability to estimate time or the error rate in problem-solving, also exhibit a circadian periodicity.

Of more practical importance are the recent studies showing that responses of the organism to drugs and other diverse insults may be very

* In a recent publication a membrane model has been proposed:

Njus, D., F. M. Sulzman, and J. W. Hastings. Membrane model for the circadian clock. Nature 248:116–120, 1974.

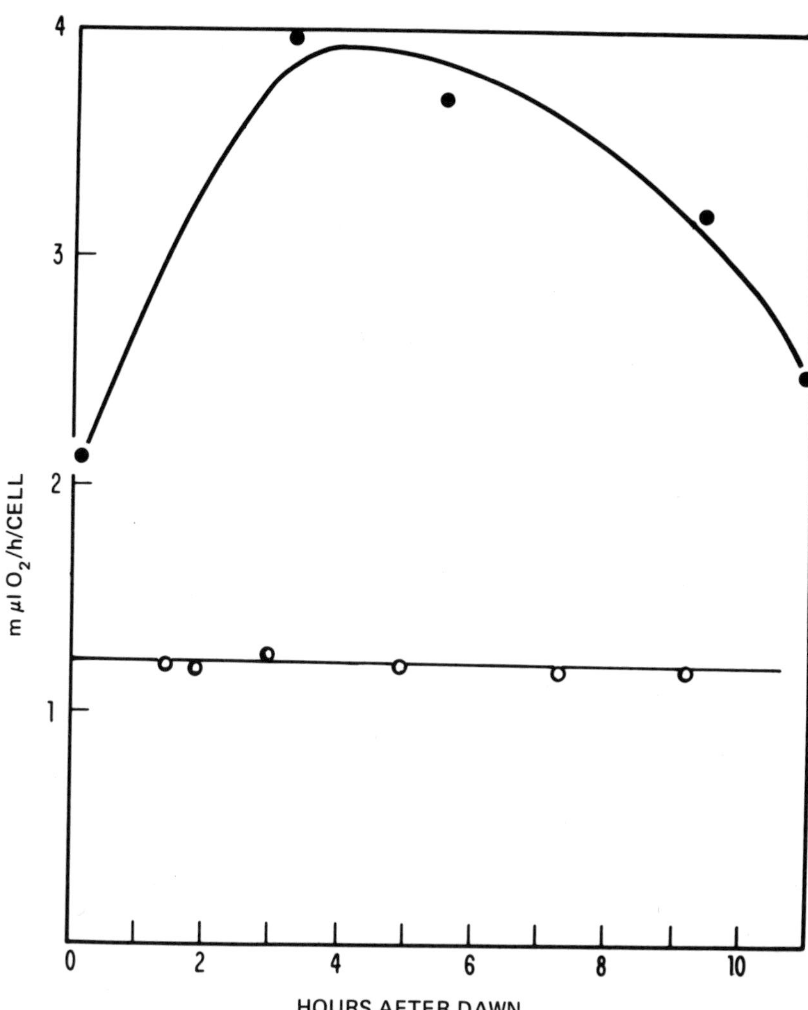

FIGURE 5 Measurement of the photosynthetic capacity in single isolated cells of *Gonyaulax* from a culture grown in light:dark 12:12 conditions before transfer to continuous light. Cells kept in dim light (50 ft-c) exhibit a rhythm (solid circles) whereas those kept in bright light (800 ft-c) do not (open circles). The absolute levels of photosynthesis are not comparable under the two conditions. (From Sweeney.[25] Copyright 1961 by Cold Spring Harbor Laboratory, Cold Spring Harbor, N.Y.)

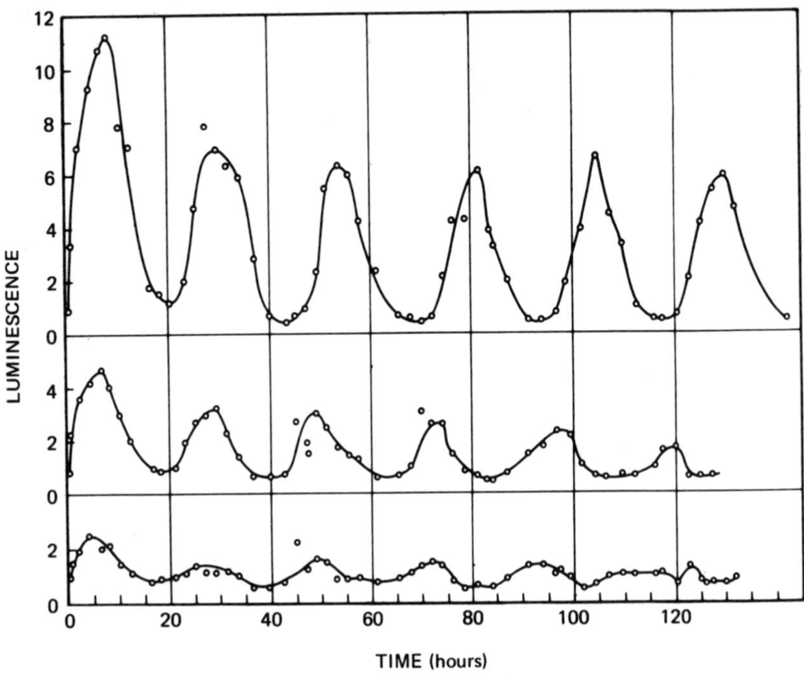

FIGURE 6 This experiment illustrates the effect of light intensity upon the period. The cells were grown in light:dark 12:12 conditions (800 ft-c during the light period). The beginning of the experiment, shown on the graph as 0 time, fell at the end of a normal light period. At this time, cells were placed in constant light at different intensities, as noted. The period in hours, also noted, is a function of light intensity. No rhythm can be measured at a very bright intensity. Luminescence in arbitrary units. (After Hastings.[14])

different at different times of day.[22] Some of these have been summarized in graphic form by Aschoff (Figure 7). Halberg [11] and his associates demonstrated many years ago that mice are far more susceptible to killing by ethanol at one time of day than at another; similar results have been obtained for other agents, such as ouabain and endotoxin. The finding that whole-body x-irradiation is far more effective in killing at one time of day caused a considerable stir when reported, but it now appears well verified. Similar rhythms in sensitivity (for example, skin reactions to histamine) are known in man.

A study of circadian phenomena in man requires that time cues be excluded, whether they are in the form of light–dark cycles or in some other form. Only then can we be reasonably sure that we are observing

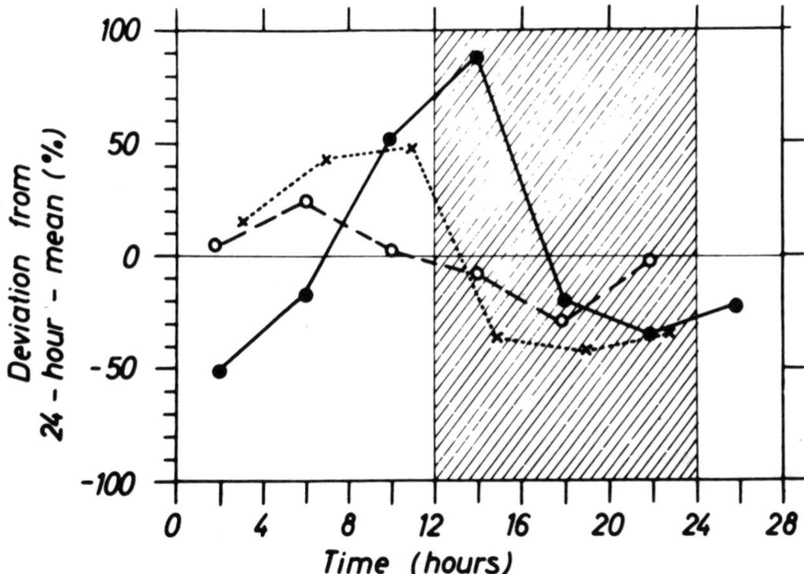

FIGURE 7 Rhythms of responsiveness to stimuli or drugs in mice kept in artificial light:dark cycles (shaded darkness). Open circles indicate duration of narcosis after pentobarbitol, the crosses time to death after whole-body irradiation, and the solid circles, mortality from a dose of ethanol. (From Aschoff.[2])

the properties of the clock, and only then can we isolate and study individually various factors, including zeitgebers. The most extensive and important experiments on human circadian rhythms have been carried out by Professor J. Aschoff and his colleagues at the Max-Planck Institute in Erling-Andechs, Germany. There they have built special underground bunkers with sophisticated facilities for such experiments, where human subjects can live in complete isolation for long periods—3 or 4 weeks. From these studies (Figure 2), it is known that human subjects exhibit a circadian day, and that they are also subject to entrainment and phase shifting. Entrainment of the circadian system to 24 h not only results in adjustment to the environmental periodicity of light, temperature, and so on; it also provides a temporal order within the organism. The physiology of the "disordered" state is not well described. It may be that time shifting (as after a transoceanic trip) may be a model for this. Or in a *non*entrained individual, internal desynchronization, which is probably deleterious in the long run, may occur (Figure 8); thus far, however, evidence for this has been found only in plants.

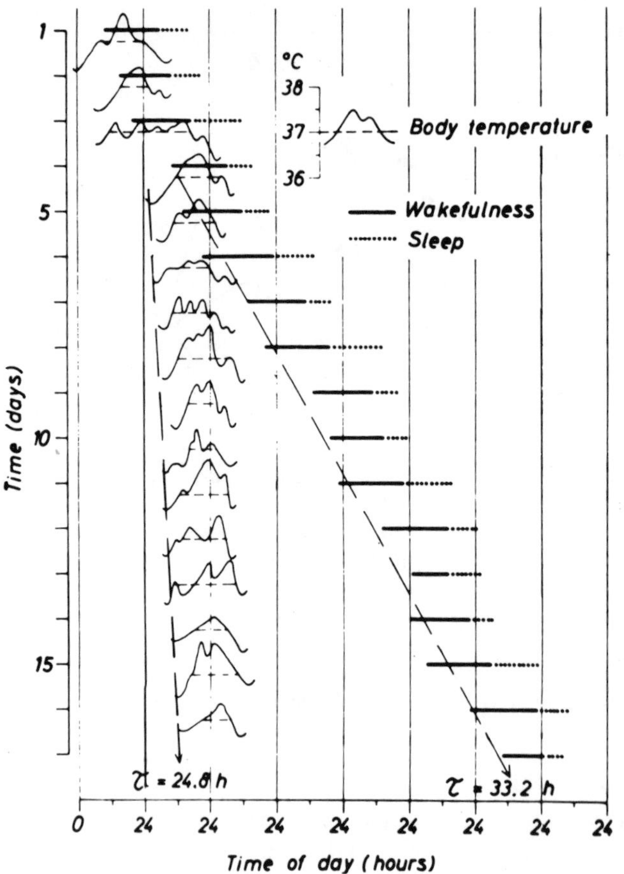

FIGURE 8 Dissociation of rhythms of rectal temperature and of activity of a human subject enclosed in isolation without time cues. Consecutive periods are shown as horizontal lines. Note that the rectal-temperature rhythm has a circadian period, close to 24 h, and that the activity rhythm is far different. (From Aschoff.[2])

The Newborn

Much less is known about rhythms in neonates. Among the laboratories where this is being investigated are those of Dr. Theodore Hellbrügge in Munich and Dr. Arthur C. Parmelee at the University of California, Los Angeles. Although circadian rhythms are viewed as innate, they are apparently not present at birth, and appear only after several weeks. Only in the premature is there something like a 24-hour rhythm. But this rhythm soon disappears, and later on, as in the full-term newborn, the circadian system emerges and is later entrained to 24 h.

Perspectives and Protocols

From the above facts and considerations one might easily conclude that the newborn should be subjected to entraining conditions as promptly as possible. But, in fact, how sure are we that light–dark cycles constitute the zeitgeber for entrainment in infants? From animal studies it seemed clear that light is *the* zeitgeber. But recent unpublished studies of Aschoff have shown that other factors—sound and social signals, for example—are of equal or greater importance in human adults. Therefore, feeding schedules, handling, noise, and so on may be sufficient or even better for the entrainment of the developing circadian system.

For phototherapy a 24-hour bright–dim light schedule could be devised (16 h bright, 8 h dim) in which the total exposure would be not much less than with continuous light. The same effect might be achieved by "skeleton" periods; for example, two 1-hour periods of darkness at approximately dawn and dusk could be used.

Light for phototherapy might also be more effective at one time of day than at another, as it is in photosynthesis in some organisms (Figure 5). This should be investigated. However, there may be *some* time-related process that would result in an alternating cycle of effectiveness. For example, such a cycle might be based on the rhythm of approximately 2 h that appears first in newborns. Perhaps a 20-minute exposure to light followed by a 100-minute dark period is equal in effectiveness to continuous light. If we extend this idea to the molecular level, it is possible that the photochemical step in phototherapy is much faster than the subsequent dark reactions. Light absorbed in 1/1000 of a second might be sufficient to keep dark reactions saturated for 10 or 100 times that length of time. Total irradiation could thereby be reduced by a factor of 10 or 100.

Such questions merit full exploration in experimental phototherapy in future years.

REFERENCES

1. Aschoff, J. Circadian rhythms in man. Science 148:1427–1432, 1965.
2. Aschoff, J. Desynchronization and resynchronization of human circadian rhythms, pp. 1–11. In AGARD Conference Proceedings, No. 25, Behavioral Problems in Aerospace Medicine. London: Technical Editing and Reproduction, 1967.

3. Aschoff, J., Ed. Circadian Clocks. Amsterdam: North-Holland Publishing Co., 1965. 479 pp.
4. Biological clocks. Cold Spring Harbor Symp. Quant. Biol. 25:1–524, 1960.
5. Bünning, E. The Physiological Clock. (Rev. 3rd ed.) New York: Springer-Verlag, 1973. 256 pp.
6. Bünning, E., and I. Moser. Influence of valinomycin on circadian leaf movements of *Phaseolus*. Proc. Natl. Acad. Sci. (USA) 69:2732–2733, 1972.
7. Colquhoun, W. P., Ed. Biological Rhythms and Human Performance. London and New York: Academic Press, Inc., 1971. 350 pp.
8. Ehret, C. F., and E. Trucco. Molecular models for the circadian clock. I. The chronon concept. J. Theor. Biol. 15:240–262, 1967.
9. Enright, J. T. The internal clock of drunken isopods. Z. Vergl. Physiol. 75: 332–346, 1971.
10. Goodwin, B. C. Temporal Organizations in Cells: A Dynamic Theory of Cellular Control Processes. New York: Academic Press, Inc., 1963. 163 pp.
11. Halberg, F. Chronobiology. Ann. Rev. Physiol. 31:675–725, 1969.
12. Harker, J. E. The Physiology of Diurnal Rhythms. London: Cambridge University Press, 1964. 114 pp.
13. Hastings, J. W. Biochemical mechanisms involved in biological rhythms and cycles, pp. 127–140. In J. de Ajuriaguerra, Ed. Cycles Biologiques et Psychiatrie: Third Bel-Air Symposium, Genève, Septembre, 1967. Geneva: Georg et Cie SA, 1968.
14. Hastings, J. W. The role of light in persistent daily rhythms, pp. 333–361. In A. C. Giese, Ed. Photophysiology. Vol. 1. General Principles: Action of Light on Plants. New York: Academic Press, Inc., 1964.
15. Hastings, J. W., and B. M. Sweeney. On the mechanism of temperature independence in a biological clock. Proc. Natl. Acad. Sci. (USA) 43:804–811, 1957.
16. Luce, G. G. Biological Rhythms in Human and Animal Physiology. New York: Dover Publications, Inc., 1971. 183 pp.
17. Mills, J. N. Human circadian rhythms. Physiol. Rev. 46:128–171, 1966.
18. Pavlidis, T. Biological Oscillators: Their Mathematical Analysis. New York: Academic Press, Inc., 1973.
19. Chance, B., E. K. Pye, A. K. Ghosh, and B. Hess, Ed. Biological and Biochemical Oscillators. New York: Academic Press, Inc., 1973.
20. Pittendrigh, C. S. On temporal organization in living systems. Harvey Lect. 56:93–125, 1961.
21. Rawson, K. S. Experimental modification of mammalian endogenous activity rhythms, pp. 791–800. In R. B. Withrow, Ed. Photoperiodism and Related Phenomena in Plants and Animals. Washington, D.C.: American Association for the Advancement of Science, 1959.
22. Reinberg, A., and F. Halberg. Circadian chronopharmacology. Ann. Rev. Pharmacol. 11:455–492, 1971.
23. Richter, C. P. Biological Clocks in Medicine and Psychiatry. Springfield, Ill.: Charles C Thomas Co., 1965. 119 pp.
24. Sweeney, B. M. Rhythmic Phenomena in Plants (Experimental Botany Monographs, Vol. 3). New York: Academic Press, Inc., 1969. 147 pp.
25. Sweeney, B. M. The photosynthetic rhythm in single cells of *Gonyaulax polyedra*. Cold Spring Harbor Symp. Quant. Biol. 25:145–148, 1960.

MARSHALL H. KLAUS

Important Considerations in the Clinical Management of Infants with Hyperbilirubinemia

Nurses in the intensive care unit can barely keep up with what they are asked to do; thus, if bilirubin lights are recommended, it is important that any new duties for nurses, such as measurements of light, be kept simple.

Second, if the Committee recommends light therapy, I suggest that they prepare different recommendations for infants of various sizes and those with differing conditions.

Third, I have been interested in the effect of various elements of the environment on the infant. As you know, for the past 15–20 years, there has been tremendous interest in trying to determine how the premature infant should be heated. At present, we know at what environmental temperature there is an increased survival and at what temperature the infants grow more rapidly, but we still do not know the effect of temperature on the development of the infant at 5, 10, 15, or even 20 years.

I make this comparison with temperature, which has been intensively studied, and then ask: What about sound? What about cutaneous stimulation? And, of course, what about light?

I think it is going to be hard to say that lights are either helping or hindering development, and another difficult question then comes: What is optimum development?

I should like to describe two studies that may be relevant. One is a study by Siqueland and Lipsitt at Brown University.[8] In their intervention, which was given during the infants' entire hospital stay, half of the premature infants were stimulated by being picked up and talked to for 20 minutes a day. The control group was not given any additional stimulation. The infants were brought back at 4 months and studied by observers who did not know which group the infants were in, and they were tested to determine the infants' ability to focus a camera. When the infant sucked at a certain rate, the picture came into focus. About 75 percent of the infants who were given increased stimulation were able to focus the picture, but only 20 percent of the nonstimulated premature infants could accomplish this task.

Just joggling a premature infant for about 20 minutes a day will increase his weight gain.[1] Other investigators have touched a baby 5 minutes every hour and markedly changed stool habits and activity pattern.[2] Immature infants may be much more sensitive in the first day or two to any environmental change.

The difficult decision is: What should we consider to be good? Is it good to be able to focus a camera? It is a knotty problem to know what type of light is best for the human infant. It is a difficult question, and it is going to keep everyone busy for a long time.

I should like to raise another issue, which is simpler. There is a second patient that we all take care of, and this is the mother. Blue lights are extremely frightening and disturbing to the mother. About 30–40 percent of all battered children are premature infants.[4] Also, about 25–40 percent of all infants who come into a children's hospital with failure to thrive without organic disease (this is a disease that accounts for about 2–3 percent of all admissions to children's hospitals) were sick as neonates or were prematures.[7] In such diseases there are problems of attachment of mother to infant. It is possible that some of these problems are produced by the hospital. Blue bilirubin lights can be extremely upsetting since they make the infant appear dead. Mothers who have sick or premature infants quickly believe the infants will die even without bilirubin lights and start anticipatory grief (the process of giving up the infant).[3, 4] For this reason, it is important not to use lights with only the blue spectrum.

A fourth recommendation is related to eye patches. There is accumulating evidence that human mothers make significant attachments to infants in the first minutes and hours of life, and this attachment occurs in part when the mother looks at the infant's eyes.[5, 6] As you know, the infant can see and follow and has visual preferences (which change during the first year of life). The infant has the visual apparatus to follow and see the mother at a distance of 12 in.

If you use phototherapy and patches on the infant's eyes, the mother may have a difficult time making an attachment to the infant. We have found that when you first present a mother with her baby without patches and record everything she says, 80 percent of the verbal content is related to the eyes: "Please open your eyes. Open your eyes. If you open your eyes, I will know you are alive." [5] I have sometimes heard mothers say, "But then the baby looked at me, and I thought he liked me; I then became fond of him." If you patch the eyes, you prevent or quench (if you wish to use a chemical term) mother-to-infant attachment at that visit.

I have seen eye patches fall over the infant's nose and obstruct the nostrils. Since an infant is an obligate nose breather, the eye patches can obstruct respiration. Although they are necessary, they almost asphyxiated one of our own low-birth-weight newborns when they dropped over his nose.

It is my personal prejudice that some diseases, and here I refer to battering and failure to thrive, are produced in part by the hospital and particularly by equipment, such as phototherapy equipment. I strongly urge that when a mother visits, the lights be turned off and the eye patches removed from the baby. I am much more sure of this than I am about how much light a baby should have.

REFERENCES

1. Freedman, D., H. Boverman, and N. Freedman. Effects of Kinesthetic Stimulation on Weight Gain and on Smiling in the Premature Infants. Paper presented at meeting of the American Orthopsychiatry Association, San Francisco, April 1966.
2. Hasselmeyer, E. G. Handling and Premature Infant Behavior. Ann Arbor, Mich: University Microfilms, Inc., 1963.
3. Kaplan, D. M., and E. A. Mason. Maternal reactions to premature birth viewed as an acute emotional disorder. Am. J. Orthopsychiatr. 30:539–552, 1960.
4. Klaus, M. H., and A. A. Fanaroff. Care of the High-Risk Neonate. Philadelphia: W. B. Saunders Co., 1973. 358 pp.
5. Klaus, M. H., J. H. Kennell, N. Plumb, and S. Zuehlke. Human maternal behavior at the first contact with her young. Pediatrics 46:187–192, 1970.
6. Robson, K. S. The role of eye-to-eye contact in maternal–infant attachment. J. Child Psychol. Psychiatr. 8:13–25, 1967.
7. Shaheen, E., D. Alexander, M. Truskowsky, and G. J. Barbero. Failure to thrive—A retrospective profile. Clin. Pediatr. 7:255–261, 1968.
8. Siqueland, E., and L. Lipsitt. Learning ability and its enhancement, pp. 52–55. In J. Henkes and R. Schain, Eds. Learning Disorders in Children. Report of the 61st Ross Conference on Pediatric Research. Columbus: Ross Laboratories, 1971.

Contributors

ROBERT J. ANDERSON, Beckman Instruments, Inc., Fullerton, Calif.

COLIN S. BERRY, University of Pennsylvania Medical Division, Veterans Administration Hospital, Philadelphia

THOMAS R. BOGGS, JR., Department of Pediatrics, University of Pennsylvania Medical School, Philadelphia, and Section on Newborn Pediatrics, Pennsylvania Hospital, Philadelphia

MARILYN L. COWGER, Department of Pediatrics, Albany Medical College of Union University, Albany, N.Y.

CHRISTOPHER S. FOOTE, Department of Chemistry, University of California, Los Angeles

J. W. HASTINGS, Biological Laboratories, Harvard University, Cambridge, Mass.

LOIS JOHNSON, Department of Pediatrics, University of Pennsylvania Medical School, Philadelphia, and Section on Newborn Pediatrics, Pennsylvania Hospital, Philadelphia

MARSHALL H. KLAUS, Department of Pediatrics, Case Western Reserve School of Medicine, and Director of Newborn Nurseries, Rainbow Babies & Childrens Hospital, Cleveland, Ohio

DAVID A. LIGHTNER, Department of Chemistry, University of Nevada, Reno

ANTONY F. MCDONAGH, Department of Medicine, University of California, San Francisco

GERARD B. ODELL, Department of Pediatrics, Johns Hopkins Hospital, Baltimore, Md.

J. DONALD OSTROW, University of Pennsylvania Medical Division, Veterans Administration Hospital, Philadelphia

JOHANNA S. SCHRUBEN, Optics, R&D, Westinghouse Research Laboratories, Pittsburgh, Pa.

THOMAS P. VOGL, Department of Pediatrics, College of Physicians and Surgeons, Columbia University, New York

PAUL Y. K. WU, Department of Pediatrics, University of Southern California School of Medicine, and the Los Angeles County-USC Medical Center

RICHARD J. WURTMAN, Department of Nutrition and Food Science (Endocrinology and Metabolism), Massachusetts Institute of Technology, Cambridge

JOHN E. ZAREMBO, Analytical and Physical Chemistry Division, Smith, Kline and French Laboratories, Philadelphia, Pa.